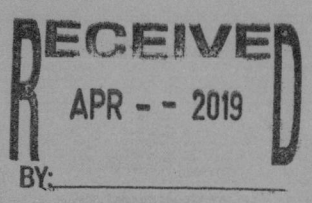

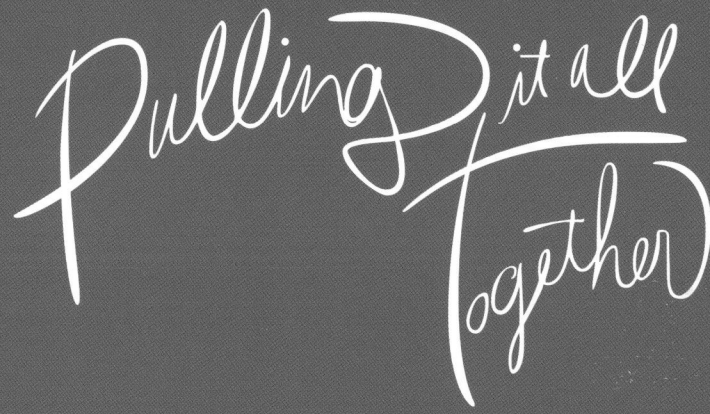

Pulling It All Together

ESSENTIAL STYLE ADVICE
ON BEING BEAUTIFUL,
CONFIDENT & (MOST OF ALL)
happy!

PAUL WHARTON

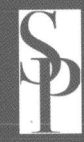

Skyhorse Publishing

Skyhorse Publishing books may be purchased in bulk at special discounts for sales promotion, corporate gifts, fund-raising, or educational purposes. Special editions can also be created to specifications. For details, contact the Special Sales Department, Skyhorse Publishing, 307 West 36th Street, 11th Floor, New York, NY 10018 or info@skyhorsepublishing.com.

Skyhorse® and Skyhorse Publishing® are registered trademarks of Skyhorse Publishing, Inc.®, a Delaware corporation.

Visit our website at www.skyhorsepublishing.com.

10 9 8 7 6 5 4 3 2 1

Library of Congress Cataloging-in-Publication Data is available on file.

Interior book design by Aidah Fontenot
Logo design by Michael Woestehoff
Cover photo by Chris Mills

Print ISBN: 978-1-5107-2234-7
Ebook ISBN: 978-1-5107-2235-4

Printed in China

Note: Before undertaking any exercise, using recipes, products or suggestions set out in this book, please consult a medical professional to ensure that you have no allergies, injuries, or conditions that may be exacerbated by any of these steps. Exercise and food references in this book are illustrative only and may not be suitable for all people. Please diet and exercise responsibly.

TO
MY DEAR

Mother, Brenda Herian, and father, Paul Wharton Sr., thank you for encouraging me to continue to try again each time I was discouraged. The love you've shown me will never be forgotten. To Cynthia Wilson, thank you for being one of the first people to believe I had something special to offer the world. To Holly, Anasia, Nadia, and Seana, you are the best cheerleaders a brother and uncle could have. And to my dearest friends, Jemaja, Timothais, Sidra, and Mikail, my life wouldn't be nearly as joy-filled or pulled together without your friendship. I love you to the moon and back.

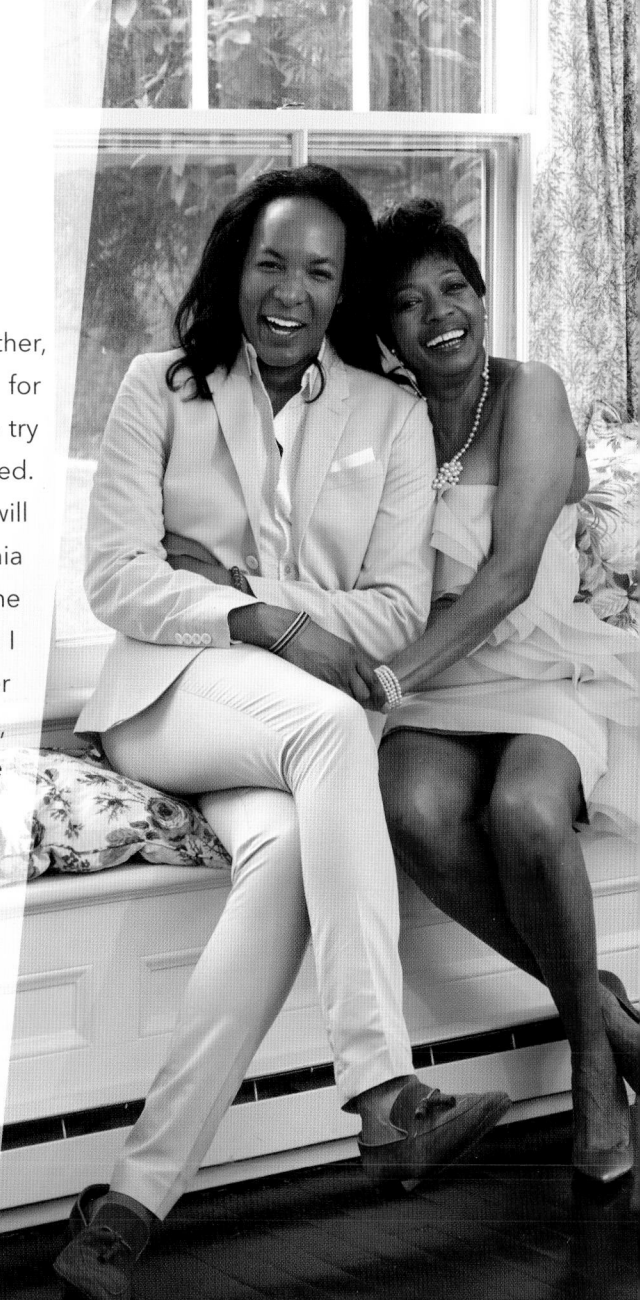

TABLE OF CONTENTS

I'VE BEEN INTRIGUED

by the story of Edith "Big Edie" Bouvier Beale and her daughter Edith "Little Edie" Bouvier Beale since I saw the 2009 HBO original film "Grey Gardens," starring Drew Barrymore and Jessica Lange. I immediately set out to find the 1975 documentary film and other materials to learn more about the aunt and cousin of Jackie Kennedy Onassis and exactly what transpired in their lifetimes. As life would have it, years later I would become friends with the home's owners, Sally Quinn, Ben Bradlee, and their son Quinn (who married my close friend Pari). Ben passed away in 2014 and since then, things were never quite the same at Grey Gardens for Sally. In the summer of 2017, Sally extended an offer for my Mother and I to vacation at Grey Gardens. I was in the process of finishing this book and thought why not take my manuscript and my Mom to East Hampton for an inspired vacation where we'd make amazing food and a lifetime of memories. Photographer Barry Harley came along with his wife Julie, as well as my friend Rebecca James from NYC to help us recreate some iconic Bouvier Beale shots and enjoy the beautiful home and gardens. Every night after dinner, I headed up to Sally's writing room, which overlooks the pool and beautiful gardens. I'd pop open my laptop and go to work, sending pages to my editor Mikail Chowdhury for review. On the final evening, as I was rounding out the last chapter and before I took my evening walk around Grey Gardens, I received a note from Mikail, "Job well done, mate. Your book is complete." I was elated! As I finished my celebratory libation, I felt thankful for creativity and guidance, and I raised my glass to "Big and Little Edie" and to Sally Quinn for sharing the magic of Grey Gardens with me. I've used several images from our time at Grey Gardens throughout this book. My hope is that *Pulling It All Together* serves as a source of inspiration and motivation to you, just as Grey Gardens did for me.

LOVE, PAUL

THE GREY GARDENS CONNECTION

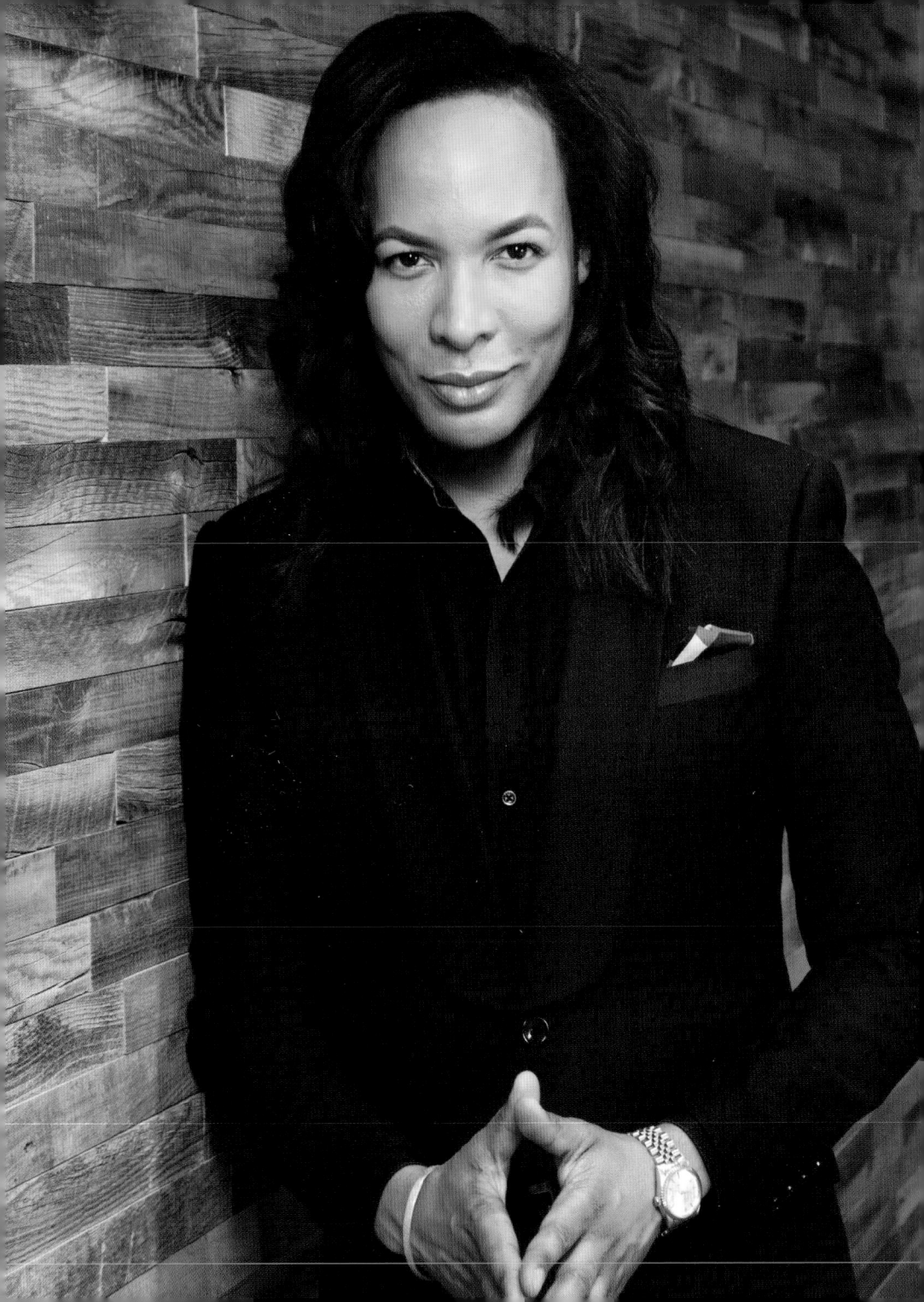

MOST OF US REMEMBER

the first time we felt our look wasn't totally pulled together. For me it was sitting in my sixth-grade classroom at James H. Harrison Elementary School in Laurel, Maryland. I'd known picture day was coming for months and rejoiced in fantasizing about my supremely stylish picture day outfit. I couldn't wait to see the look on the faces of Eric Globerman, Nicole Girard, Chris Horn, and my other classmates when I whisked into the classroom with my fresh-off-the-rack, perfectly coordinated designer duds and carefully coiffed hair. I was going to take the best picture in the school (possibly even in the state of Maryland) and everyone would clamor for a signed copy of my picture. My photograph would set the standard for all picture days across the county for generations to come.

Oh yes, this all happened in my head! Two weeks before picture day, I mentioned to my mother that I wanted her to start looking for new outfits for me when she went to the mall. She may or may not have heard me, but I wasn't overly concerned because I was lucky and my mom bought me new clothes often. Another week went by, no new additions to my closet were noted, but I still had time. The week of picture day was very busy for me. I had a new Sega video game and instead of asking my mom again about a new outfit or planning something nice to wear from what I already had, I decided to fully dedicate myself to my latest video game. After staying up way past my bedtime mastering my Sega—and sneaking two pieces of pecan pie out of the kitchen at around midnight—the morning of picture day finally arrived.

I slept right through my alarm, and when I finally came to from my sugar binge I didn't even have enough time to take a shower, put a drop of product in my hair, nor had I selected or ironed an outfit. In fact, I was in such a haze from the pie and late-night gaming session that it was all I could do to pull out a pair of wrinkly jeans and a faded T-shirt. As I ran to school I fought back the tears as I realized that my dream of picture day supremacy would not become a reality. When it was my turn in front of the camera, I almost collapsed from disappointment. (No, I did not become this dramatic later in life; it's obviously who I've always been!) I took the worst picture in history and felt awful about it.

From that moment on, I vowed to take a little more time each day to pull myself together. In a few short months, it was time for sixth-grade graduation and I showed up in the school gym looking like a cross between James Bond Jr. and a Calvin Klein kid model. I had carefully planned my outfit, which consisted of a sleek tuxedo that I tailored myself, a crisp white shirt, and bright red bow tie. My shoes were perfectly shined, and not a hair was out of place. I felt strong, confident, and totally pulled together.

THROUGHOUT MY CAREER

on television, hosting events, and working with the public, my most phenomenal triumphs have occurred when I felt that I had everything together on the outside as well as on the inside. I truly believe that when you take the time to get your look right, it frees up your mind to think more clearly and focus on what's in front of you. Your subconscious doesn't focus on your appearance, so you can exhale and feel free to be more kind, gracious, and magnanimous. Once you are pulled together, you can go about the business of achieving whatever you have set your mind to without distraction.

This book is full of my tips on how to pull together your look and your lifestyle. I hope you're able to free your mind, knowing that you are coming across as strong and confident, ready to take on extraordinary adventures and all the good things life has in store for you.

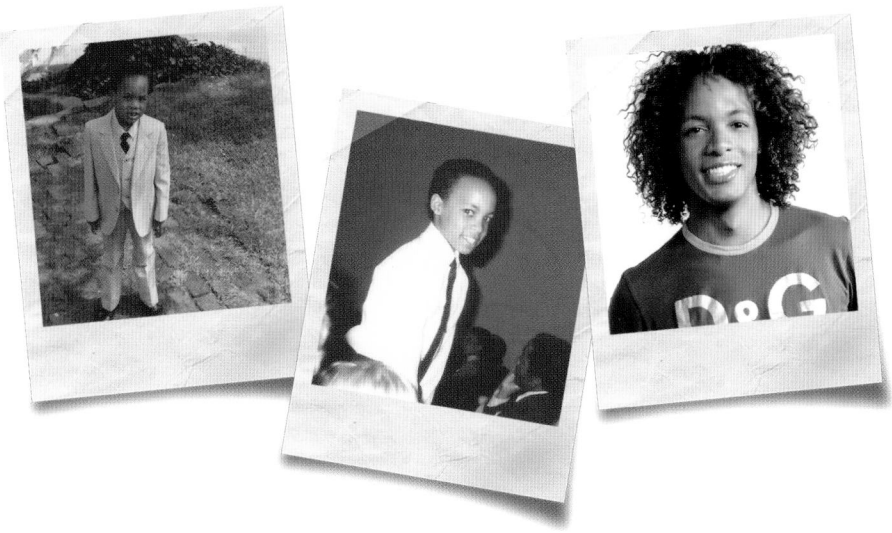

A WORD ON
PERCEPTION
& REALITY

Unless you've been stranded on a desert island with no Internet or cable, you will have seen the fashion blogs and television programs showcasing models and starlets with flawless skin, impeccable hair and makeup, and incredibly fabulous outfits with perfectly coordinated shoes and jewelry. We are bombarded with these images of perfection every day.

Most people don't realize that huge teams of professional hairstylists, makeup artists, and wardrobe stylists prepare these celebrities for their walk down the red carpet. The models in the fashion magazines also have teams of professionals preparing them for the camera, and let's not forget the special lighting, and, best of all, the process of retouching, which can remove any imperfections and even remove the appearance of additional weight from thighs or hips. On her show, *America's Next Top Model*, Tyra Banks once said that in the latter part of her career as a supermodel she didn't have to worry nearly as much about what she was eating, since a few extra pounds could easily be retouched away.

These models and celebrities don't wake up in the morning looking as flawless and fabulous as they do in those magazine spreads. They look in the mirror and see imperfections and blemishes, just like you and me.

So, how can you look like them every day? Well, the answer is, you can't, but that's because (as I explained) they don't look like that every day either.

What you can do is create the very best version of yourself. You see,

YOU ARE ALREADY PERFECT AND INCREDIBLE,

and I want you to truly believe that. By the end of this book, you are going to be celebrating how you look and know how to look your absolute best! The healthiest hair, gorgeous complexion, and clothes to complement your body type are all attainable. You may not be able to afford the expensive spas and plastic surgery procedures the stars use, but there are other alternatives, and I'm going to let you in on a few of these secrets. So, let me teach you some of the tricks that photographers and styling teams use to turn everyday women into supermodels and movie stars and show you how to feel confident every day.

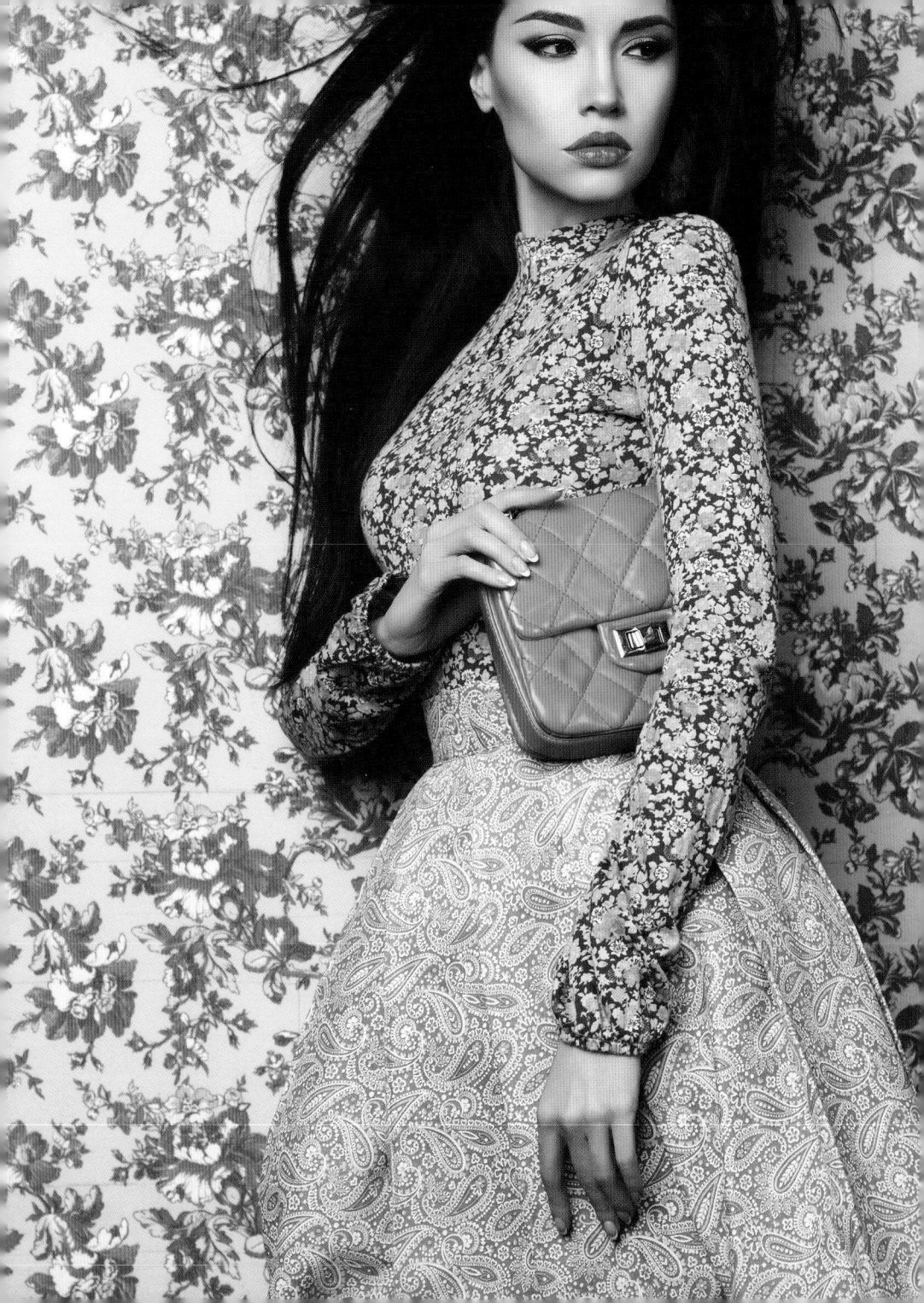

CHAPTER 1

DRESS TO IMPRESS

EVERY DAY

THE #1 RULE: CONFIDENCE

We've all heard the phrase, "It's not what you wear, but how you wear it," and now it's time to truly embrace that philosophy. In this chapter, I'll walk you through everything you need to know about clothes, from managing your closet to putting together the perfect outfit for any occasion.

The first and most important rule applies to everything in this chapter—in fact, it applies to everything you do in life—own it. Stand up straight and feel comfortable in who you are and what you have on. Trust me, it will make the difference between looking good and looking great. Be proud of who you are and how you look; this one step can change your entire appearance.

WHATEVER YOU ARE WEARING, WEAR IT WITH CONFIDENCE.

TIDINESS IS NEXT TO GODLINESS:
How to Maximize your Closet

You may be thinking, *Come on, Paul, I already know how to hang up my clothes, let's get to the shopping part*. But instead of jumping ahead, I want you to stop and think about your closet. Remember my story from the introduction? A little extra time and planning would have totally changed how my class photo turned out. Time is your most precious commodity; that's why this is important. Whether you spend your days driving your kids from school to soccer practice or are working every available hour to advance your career, we all only have twenty-four hours in each day. Following the steps here will save you at least thirty minutes (maybe even an hour) every day.

Over time, our closets become filled with clothes that we simply never wear. It's natural; we paid for something because we loved it and do not want to throw it away. But I want you to break that mindset. The key here is that if you have fewer items in a well-organized closet, you will use every single one and can get ready in half the time—no more hunting through piles of sweaters looking for the one you bought two years ago that you think would look perfect with your new jeans.

Keep it simple. Go through your closet and find any clothes with price tags still on them. (It's okay, we've all done it). Pull out anything you have not worn for over one year and anything you have only worn once. Now, go through the pile and be honest with yourself; unless you really love any of those items and will definitely use them again, give them to your local thrift store. It's okay to part with them; they're just clothes!

Now, go back to your closet and inspect the clothes that are still there. Do you have items that are really worn or faded (we all have those pants that we've worn every other day for three years and they're now fraying at the bottom) or anything that does not fit well? We'll cover the importance of how your clothes fit later in this chapter, so for now just focus on whether it is flattering on you or not. Take all those clothes out, and again be honest with yourself—anything that has seen better days or does not make you feel great when you put it on should all go to the thrift store.

Remember, you are not wasting these clothes, someone else will be able to use and love them, so let them go.

Finally, arrange the items in your closet logically; there is no magic system but as long as your pants are all in one place, your shirts in another and so on, it is fine. The key is that first thing in the morning when you are still half asleep and reach into the closet you know exactly where to go for each item.

It's that simple—these three steps will make your closet more efficient and save you real time every day.

Now on to the fun part—shopping!

BUILDING THE PERFECT WARDROBE:
How to Shop for Any Budget

Before you set foot in the mall, take a quick inventory of what you already have. Be aware of any pieces that need coordinating tops and bottoms. If you've already organized your closet, it will be easy to see what's missing.

Don't worry about your budget. I know that the models and movie stars always wear a different outfit in every paparazzi or social media shot and each one costs thousands of dollars, but here is a secret: money does not equal style, and furthermore, half the time, those clothes are borrowed or gifted to the celebrities so that people like you will notice the brands and set out to emulate the star's look. Whether you have an endless budget or a limited one, the rules are the same—you should only buy clothes that you will wear and love.

A FEW PIECES OF ADVICE TO GET YOU STARTED:

- Shop at the beginning of the season for any specific item you need for your wardrobe (your "staple" items, which we will cover later in this chapter).

- At the end of each season, shop for more high-end classic pieces that will have major markdowns like cashmere coats and simple designer pants.

- You don't need to create an entire wardrobe in one shopping trip— take your time and develop it over a season.

- While shopping, try going into different stores than you're familiar with as well as some new boutiques and department stores. We are creatures of habit and get used to one store really quickly.

- Occasionally shop with someone whose opinion you value and who you know will tell you the no-holds-barred truth. Let them choose some outfits for you that you wouldn't typically go for yourself.

- Be adventurous! There is nothing wrong with trying a different store and finding it does not work for you, but if you are bold, you may just find that perfect shop that feels like they are making things just for you.

Avoid impulse shopping! You'll only end up with odds and ends in your closet that go with nothing and do nothing but gather dust for years. Ask yourself these questions before making a purchase:

- Do you love it?
- Does it flatter you?
- Is it comfortable?
- Does it work with pieces you already have or will you have to make further purchases?
- Does it make you feel good?
- Can you afford it?

Finally, let's borrow a little advice from the men—they say that "men don't need a lot of clothes, they just need the right clothes." That is actually as true of women as of men; yes, you ladies have more options than men, but if you have too many things, it becomes overwhelming and you will not maximize your wardrobe or time. Build a great capsule wardrobe that works for you—if you love wearing pants, that's great, have a few pairs that fit you perfectly in a good range of colors, and throw a skirt in the mix just for fun sometimes. If you are a woman that loves to wear dresses, that's fine too, make sure you have a few timeless styles in black, navy, grey, white, brown, nude, and red. But if you have forty dresses, you will end up wearing the same one over and over and just ignoring everything else.

So, get yourself to the stores and shop wisely!

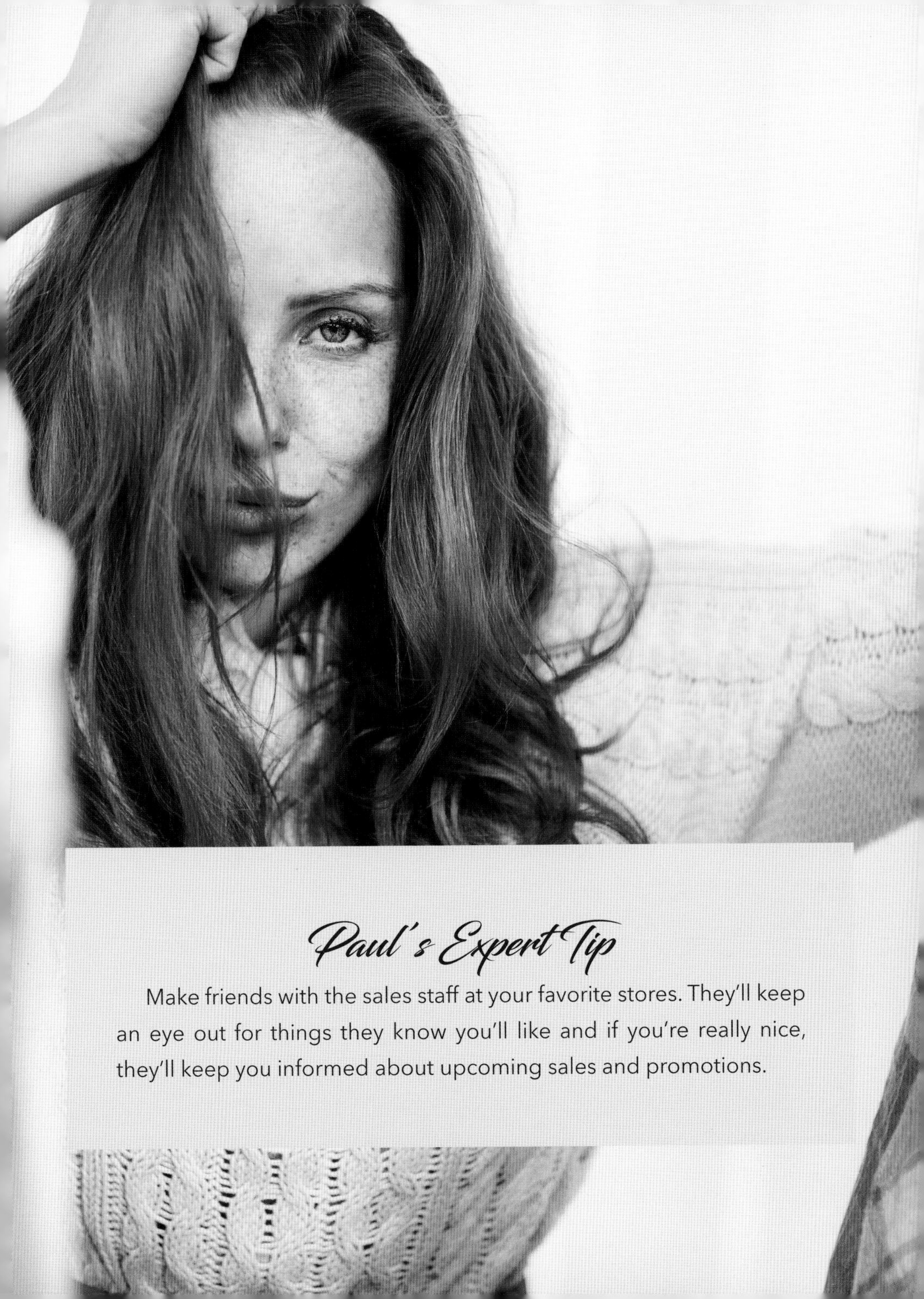

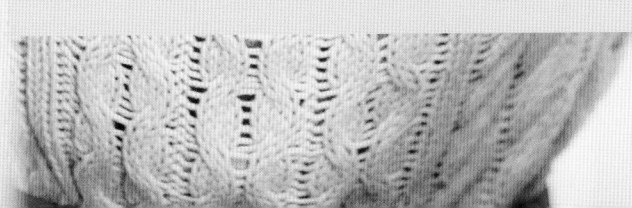

Paul's Expert Tip

Make friends with the sales staff at your favorite stores. They'll keep an eye out for things they know you'll like and if you're really nice, they'll keep you informed about upcoming sales and promotions.

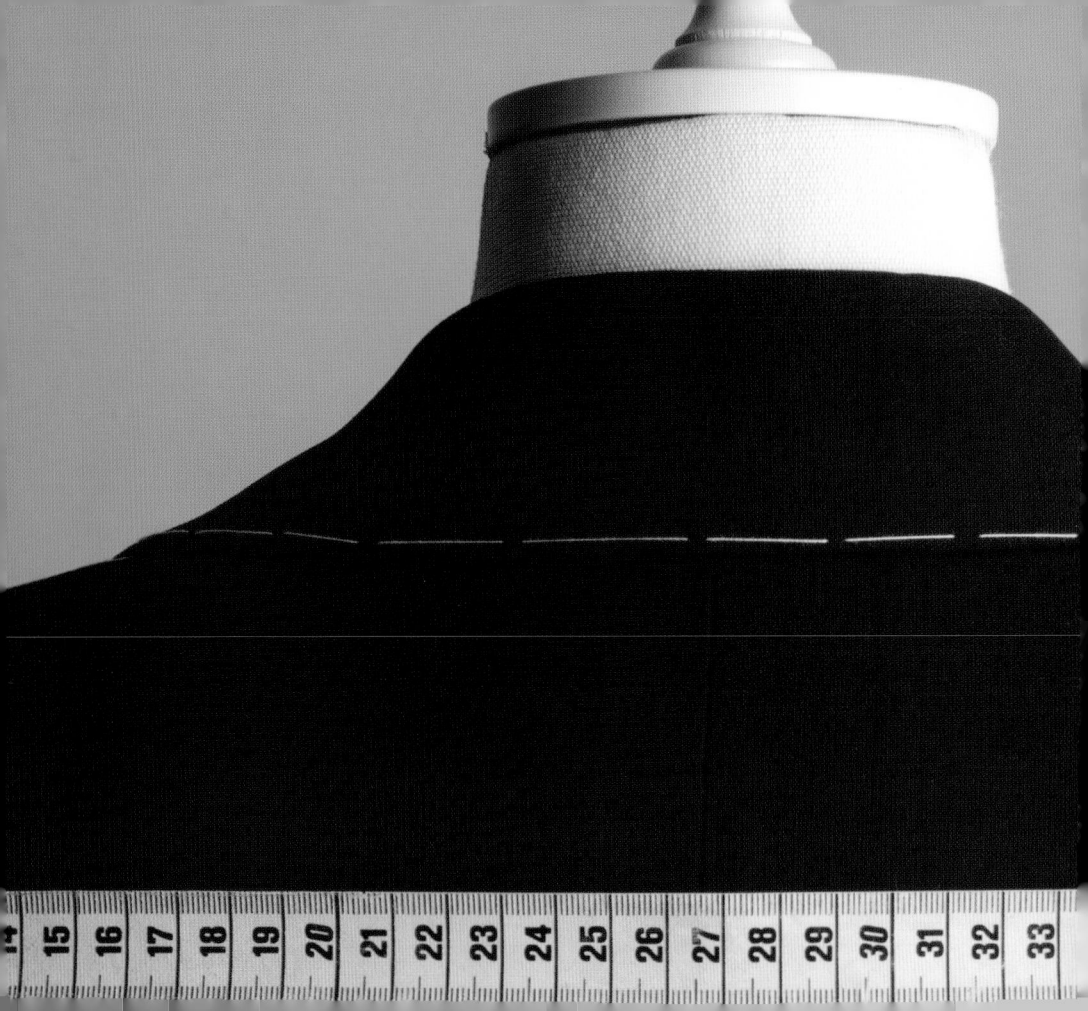

CUT
IS KING

THE IMPORTANCE OF A GOOD FIT

I've been lucky enough to live in New York City and spend time in Paris and London, cities where people really appreciate the importance of good clothes, and one thing I regularly saw is ladies heading to work and looking gorgeous even though most of them have taken the subway (or the tube/metro) into the office after having been crammed in with sweaty commuters for an hour. The key was not about their size or body shape, or even how expensive their pantsuit may have been—it was that their clothes seemed to fit them properly. When your clothes are ill-fitting, there is more of an opportunity for them to wrinkle and crease in all the wrong places.

When it comes to your wardrobe, dressing well and looking good is all about the fit. Celebrities usually look flawless because their clothes fit perfectly. They have stylists and quite often tailors to ensure that not only will their garments fit and flatter their bodies, but hide any flaws and imperfections as well. Did you know that when they do a photoshoot the stylists often use clothes pegs to pin outfits from behind to keep the fit? So again, don't aspire to look like what you see in the magazines—the stars themselves don't even look like that! But follow my steps here and I promise you will look incredible without a lot of extra effort.

Today's clothes are better cut than in the past so one should never settle for less than a perfect fit, but don't obsess over a size number. Your size will be different depending on the designer's manufacturer and store, especially with clothes marked small, medium, and large. That's why it's so important to try every piece of clothing on and to walk and sit in them before you lay down your plastic. Remember Rule #1—if you are comfortable, you will be confident.

Only buy clothes that fit and only keep clothes that fit in with the current wardrobe hanging in your closet. This way, when you open the door to your closet you'll know everything in it will fit you and your daily choices will be so much easier.

Paul's Expert Tip

Always remember, it does not matter if you have to take a bigger or smaller size or have a different cut in different stores. The art of good dressing is not about trying to hide your shape or make it look like someone else's; the art is about dressing to fit your own body. If clothes at one store don't work for you, walk away and find one that does.

SOME BASIC RULES TO FOLLOW
AS YOU SEARCH FOR THE PERFECT FIT!

Don't let shopping stress you out, take your time finding what works for you.

III Never be afraid—you should try clothing on in as many stores as you can (not all at once of course, but over time) because all stores target different customers and you have to find places that will work for you.

III Work *with* your body—no matter what size you are, any figure can be improved with clothes that fit correctly and complement your body type, so always find things that are flattering for you and make you feel good. Clothes are like a suit of armor; when you put them on you should feel powerful . . . and that power will boost your confidence.

III Every layer of an outfit is important to your overall look—if the weather is cold, don't just pile into a heavy-duty jacket, you can stay warm and be stylish by layering thicker and warmer items over a thinner base layer like a neutral T-shirt or blouse. When it gets warmer, this means you can take off a layer if it starts getting too hot and still look great.

III Choose fabrics that fall smoothly over the curves of the body and avoid fabrics that are too stiff or too clingy—clothing should skim over your body, showing the outline of your figure. It should not hug too tightly, hang, or bag too loosely. Pay close attention to fabric choices. Cheap fabrics tend to be stiffer than those of finer quality. Better quality fabrics will last longer and be more flattering on your body (Tip: if you are on a budget, it is better to have one or two quality items than five or six cheap ones).

DRESSING SLIMMER

I can't stress enough how important a good fit is to your look. Clothes too large will exaggerate your figure instead of concealing it. For example, larger women tend to buy clothes that are too big mistakenly thinking that they are hiding their flaws, when in actuality, those oversized clothes are only making them look larger. The flipside is that clothes that are too small will only emphasize problem areas and put everything you don't want people to notice on display.

A FEW GUIDELINES TO HELP YOU DRESS SLIMMER:

III The key to dressing slimmer is to create a vertical line going down—when people look at you their eyes will travel up and down and if you can emphasize this line, it will be to your advantage.

III Vertical stripes: this is an old notion, but a true one—if you're wearing vertical stripes, they naturally move the eyes up and down, giving the illusion of a slimmer look (Tip: you do not have to dress like Beetlejuice, I don't want you to go out and buy everything in a vertical pinstripe, and it does not mean that you cannot also have horizontal stripes, just keep this in mind when you are shopping).

III Single-breasted jackets will help—once again they create a vertical line whereas double-breasted jackets tend to draw the eye horizontally emphasizing breadth more than height.

III Use your assets: I am not suggesting that you wear nothing but low-cut tops or booty shorts, but don't be afraid to have clothes that fit nicely around those areas. Many women pay good money to get their curves enhanced, so whether you paid for them or not, enjoy yours!

DRESSING FOR THE SILHOUETTE YOU WANT

I know women with an athletic build who feel like they're not feminine because they don't have large breasts or a bottom. The common mistake many times is that some of these women dress for pure functionality, and wear not much more outside of sports gear and ill-fitting tops. If you are petite or skinny, my advice remains the same—own your body and make sure your clothes fit well. Here are some of my suggestions:

- As I said for dressing slimmer, you can control the way you look by understanding the way the eye moves over an outfit, so maybe try some horizontal stripes on your tops or when you wear a dress, break it up with a simple belt at the waist to enhance your silhouette and emphasize your hips.

- Double-breasted jackets can be a great and stylish addition—do not go too crazy on the shoulder pads but there is nothing wrong with playing with some power dressing styles.

- Try mixing oversized and fitted—please note that when I say "oversized," I do not mean "baggy," but just a different style of fitting. For example, try slim jeans paired with a loose-fitting blouse or T-shirt and an oversized blazer.

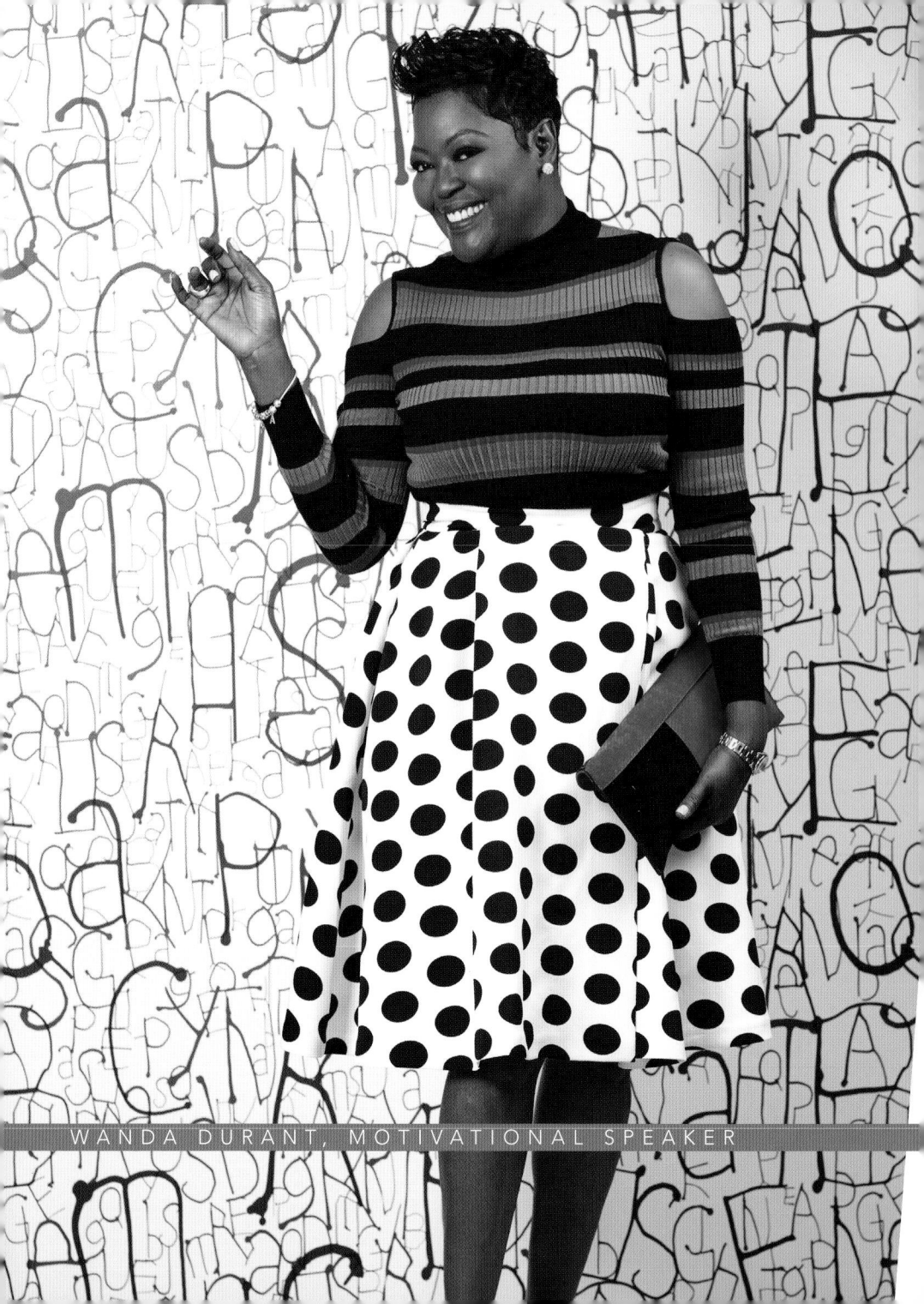
WANDA DURANT, MOTIVATIONAL SPEAKER

COLOR YOURSELF
FABULOUS
HOW TO MATCH COLORS AND
TEXTURES FOR YOUR OUTFITS

Okay, so you've established the right fit for your body and now comes time to determine what colors you look best in and purchase key pieces in those colors. Try to stick to three or four colors that coordinate with the existing pieces in your closet. Neutral colors and solids are typically the best bet for longevity—if you buy the core items in your wardrobe based on these colors, you can always match and add more daring pieces.

This is where clothes get really fun, and if you nailed the fit like I suggested earlier, you can play around with color and fabrics with confidence. I would recommend thinking about these factors when looking at color and material:

1. SIZE

Do you want to dress a little slimmer, or emphasize certain features? Color and texture can help with these. Wearing darker colors where you want to look smaller and lighter colors where you want to accentuate is one of the secrets to dressing for your size. Another is monochromatic dressing, which is the art of wearing one color or various shades of a single color from head to toe. It's very slimming because it creates a strong, unbroken line that elongates the body. Any color can be used to create this look, but darker shades such as black, navy, charcoal, chocolate, and hunter green are the most slimming and easiest to camouflage the areas of the body that you feel are less than perfect.

If you have a slimmer build and want to look more feminine, a monochromatic look with a contrasting color at any areas you want to accentuate will break up the eyeline and pick it out.

Mixing textures can add more excitement to your monochromatic outfits. Fabrics such as knits, soft suede, and leather, as well as silk and luxurious cashmere can all do just that. Matte fabrics are more slimming than shiny and embellished fabrics, just like thinner, lighter, metallic fabrics are more slimming than bulkier fabrics.

2. STATEMENT PIECES

If you've built a classic wardrobe with neutral, well-fitting items, be bold with a few statement items. Here's a simple example based on a classic outfit—let's take jeans, heeled boots, a blouse or T-shirt, and a light jacket—this is a combination that can work for everyday wear, business casual, and even semi-formal. The key to keeping it fresh is how you play with the color and textures. If you wear all black for each item, that will be a classic monochrome and if they all fit well, you will look very stylish and well-pulled together. Or you could have blue jeans, a navy top, and a cool denim jacket, throw in a pair of purple suede boots, and

Paul's Expert Tip

Invest in the best quality fabric you can afford, but if you are spending more stick with neutral colors. Quality classic fabrics will take you from season to season and year to year. Cashmere is always a great investment—it's warm, weightless, beautiful, and can be found in neutral to rich colors. Neutrals that can be mixed and matched with other classic or inexpensive trendy pieces are also essential.

you have a neutral base tone of blue with a statement of color in the boots and a different texture in the jacket. It will change the entire look.

And if you are bold with color and have lots of bright items, try the same tactic—swap one or two brighter items with a more neutral tone, or layer with a crisp white T-shirt or simple blouse and then build the color over it.

3. SKIN AND HAIR TONE

This may sound obvious, but it's incredible how little we think about it. The first tone in your outfit is your own skin color, so don't forget to work with that as well. If you have paler skin with red or light- colored hair, try contrasting your natural tone with clothes that have dark neutral shades such as navy, dark red, and grey. For those of you with a more tanned complexion or medium tone, neutrals certainly work, but maybe try some pastel shades and brighter colors as well. If you have darker skin, try it all to see what pops. Most colors should complement your skin and hair tone, so be bold.

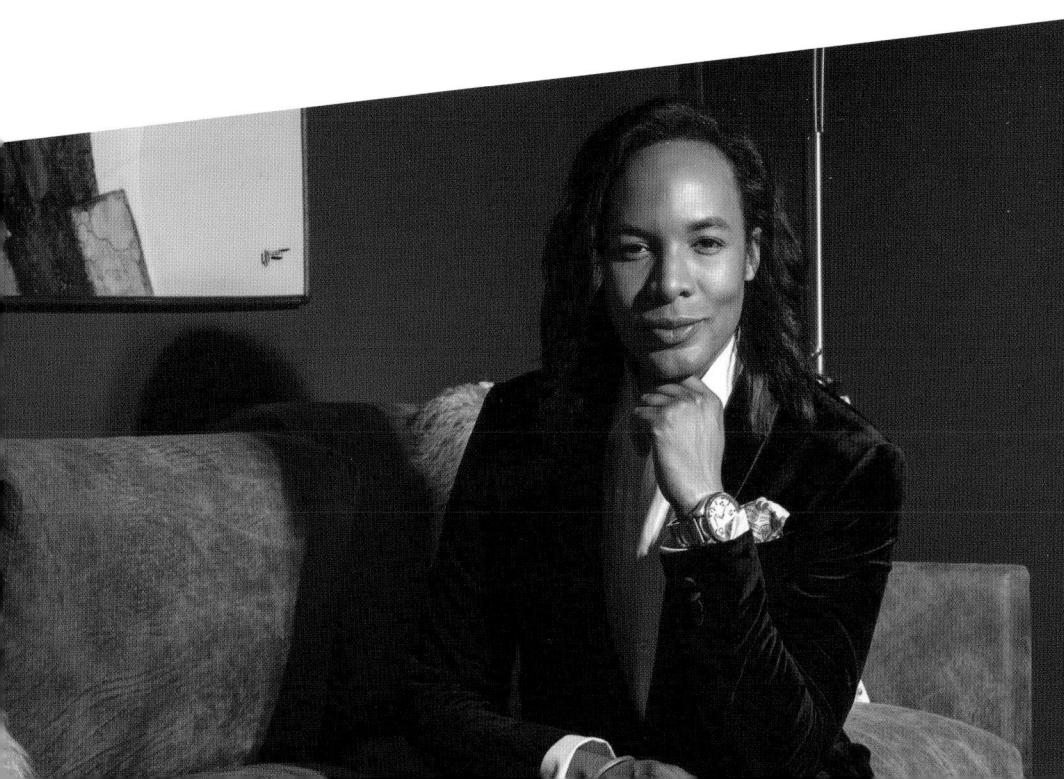

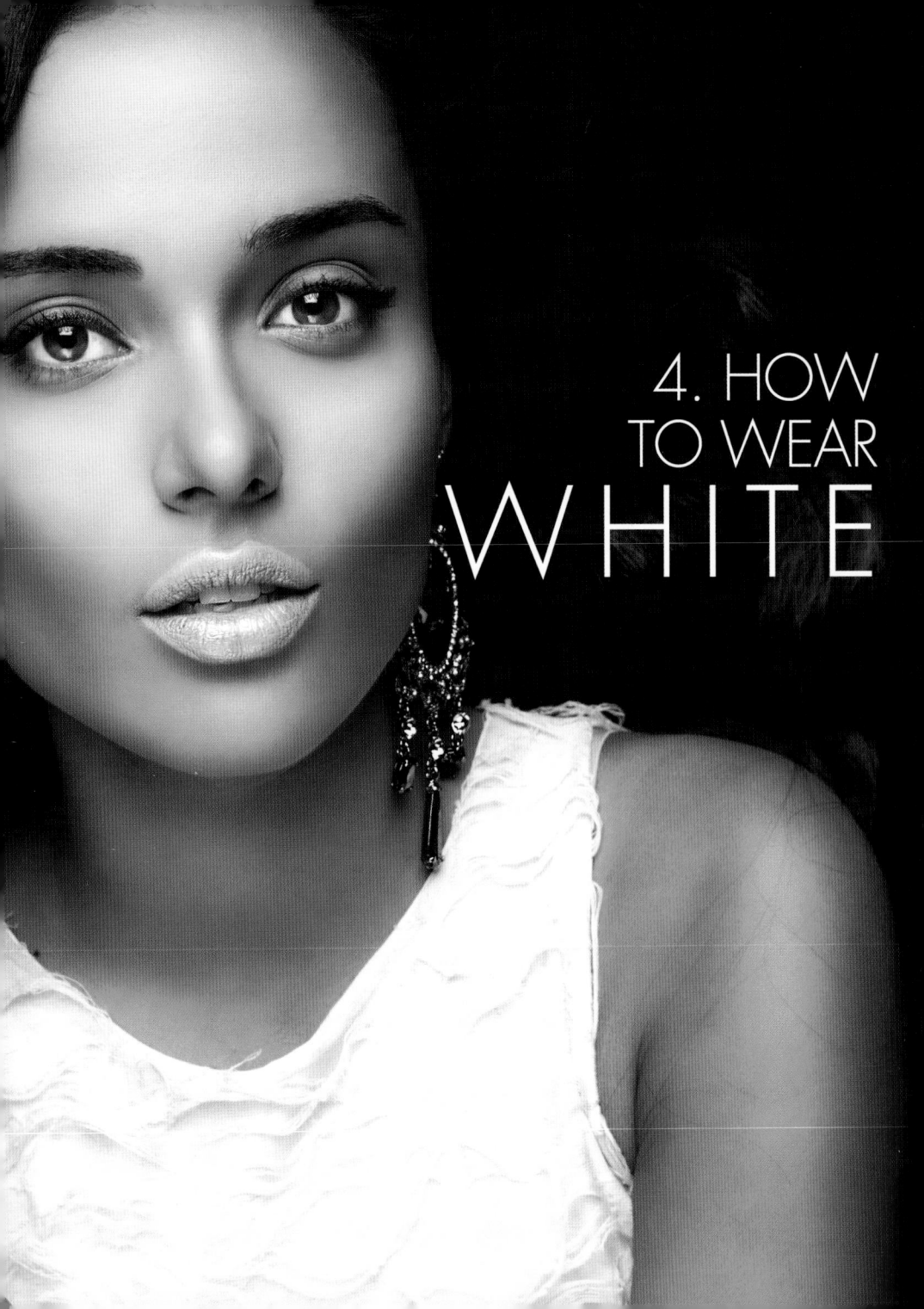

4. HOW
TO WEAR
WHITE

This may sound over the top, but trust me, white is one of the best colors you can work with and you should not be afraid of using it. Yes, it gets dirty easily, yes it's simple—but it is the ultimate classic color. A crisp white shirt will never look bad, and in one hundred years it will still be stylish. So here are my thoughts on how to pull together an outfit using this ultimate and underrated color:

- White is not just a summer color, you can wear it all year round.

- Try monochromatic head-to-toe white to elongate your body, but if you do, make sure everything is super white—don't mix in a cream or oatmeal or they'll look dingy up against your pure white.

- When wearing white, mix textures and fabrics, not color.

- White goes well with ANY color so you can have real fun with it—add color to a white outfit in unexpected ways such as a wrist full of vibrant chunky bracelets, a deep eggplant scarf, or a supple leather belt in a color that pops with a statement buckle that can be the centerpiece of your look.

- In the winter months, choose variations such as ivory, cream, beige, fawn, and off-white.

- Make sure to wear the right shoes! No black heavy pumps. Instead, opt for light, neutral tones that work better with white.

- When wearing semi-sheer white, the smartest lingerie choice is a shade closer to your skin tone. You'll be able to see the outline of your bra through your shirt unless you go with flesh-colored undergarments.

- One challenge with white pants is that it's difficult to hide any flaws, but don't be afraid to try it, just be sure to check your outfit from every angle and you can add some colorful pieces to draw attention away from any areas that you don't want focused on.

NAIL THE STAPLES:
Build A Classic Capsule Wardrobe

This is a theme I keep coming back to and I want to devote this section to focus on it. When we say "capsule wardrobe" and "staples," this does not mean you have to buy boring or dull items. But when you put together an outfit, try to imagine you are building it, like a house. You need a solid foundation, all the pieces need to fit together well, and it should make an impression no matter what the occasion.

You may be thinking, *but Paul, I can't get dressed up just to drop my kids at school and hit the grocery store*. I'm not saying you should wear a cocktail dress to attend a parent-teacher conference (not unless the other parents are trying to show you up and in that case, let them have it!), but if you have a closet stocked with good items, you never need to dress down because you will always be dressed well. Remember the ladies of New York, London, and Paris, who stagger out of a sweaty underground train and manage to look good? Not only did their clothes fit, but their outfits were usually very simply but perfectly put together; they probably have two or three combinations for work that they use over and over, five days a week, but that does not matter. They are not trying to dress for an awards show, they want to be practical and stylish.

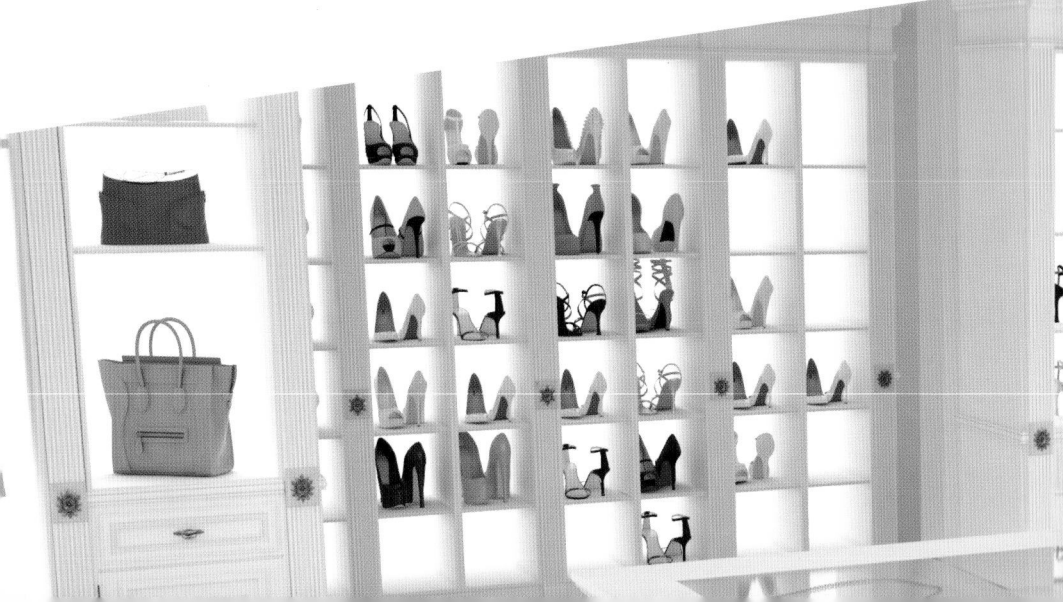

So here is the key—build a great foundation with key pieces and whether you are rushing to a business meeting or pushing a stroller with your babies, you will always look well-dressed.

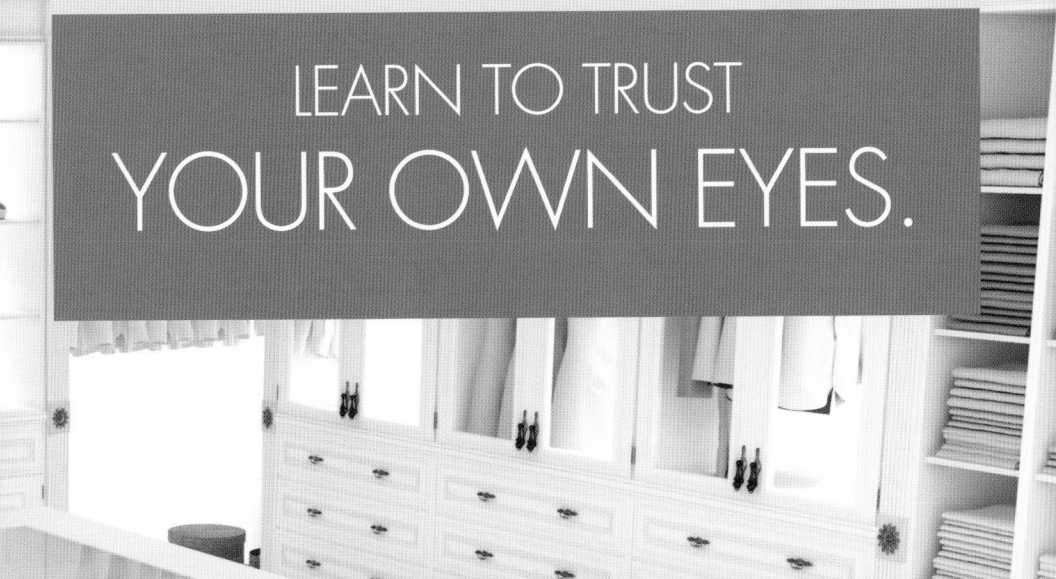

LEARN TO TRUST
YOUR OWN EYES.

JEANS

Every person has their favorite pair of jeans. They fit just right, are the perfect color, everything about them is spot on and they make you feel great. Here are a few tips to ensure every pair becomes your favorite:

III Color: start by choosing a deeper indigo hue or black for a classic look. I should not have to tell you again to make sure they fit perfectly, but remember how to use color if you want to dress for a certain body-shape—the darker the denim, the thinner you will look, lighter washes of denim and tapered legs will make you look bigger.

III Cut: try as many pairs as you need to find the perfect cut that sits nicely on your hips (they should fit without a belt) and are fitted at your bottom but comfortable enough to move and sit down in. Note that capris and cropped pants make legs look shorter so if you're petite, wear full-length trousers to create a longer line which will give you height.

III Buy your jeans a little longer than usual and have them hemmed. Specifically, you should have a pair hemmed for flats and another hemmed for heels. If necessary, use a tailor to hem your jeans to the perfect length so that it matches the rest of the denim in your wardrobe.

III To prevent your dark denims from fading and shrinking, turn them inside out and wash them in cold water. Hang your jeans to dry and finish with a warm iron.

Once you've got the right color and fit, it's all about dressing up the denim. Pair it with a silky dressy camisole. That along with a string of pearls and a pair of sexy stilettos almost always does the trick. If pearls aren't your thing, try dramatic accessories like chunky bracelets, metallic and sequinned bags, and/or long, dangly earrings.

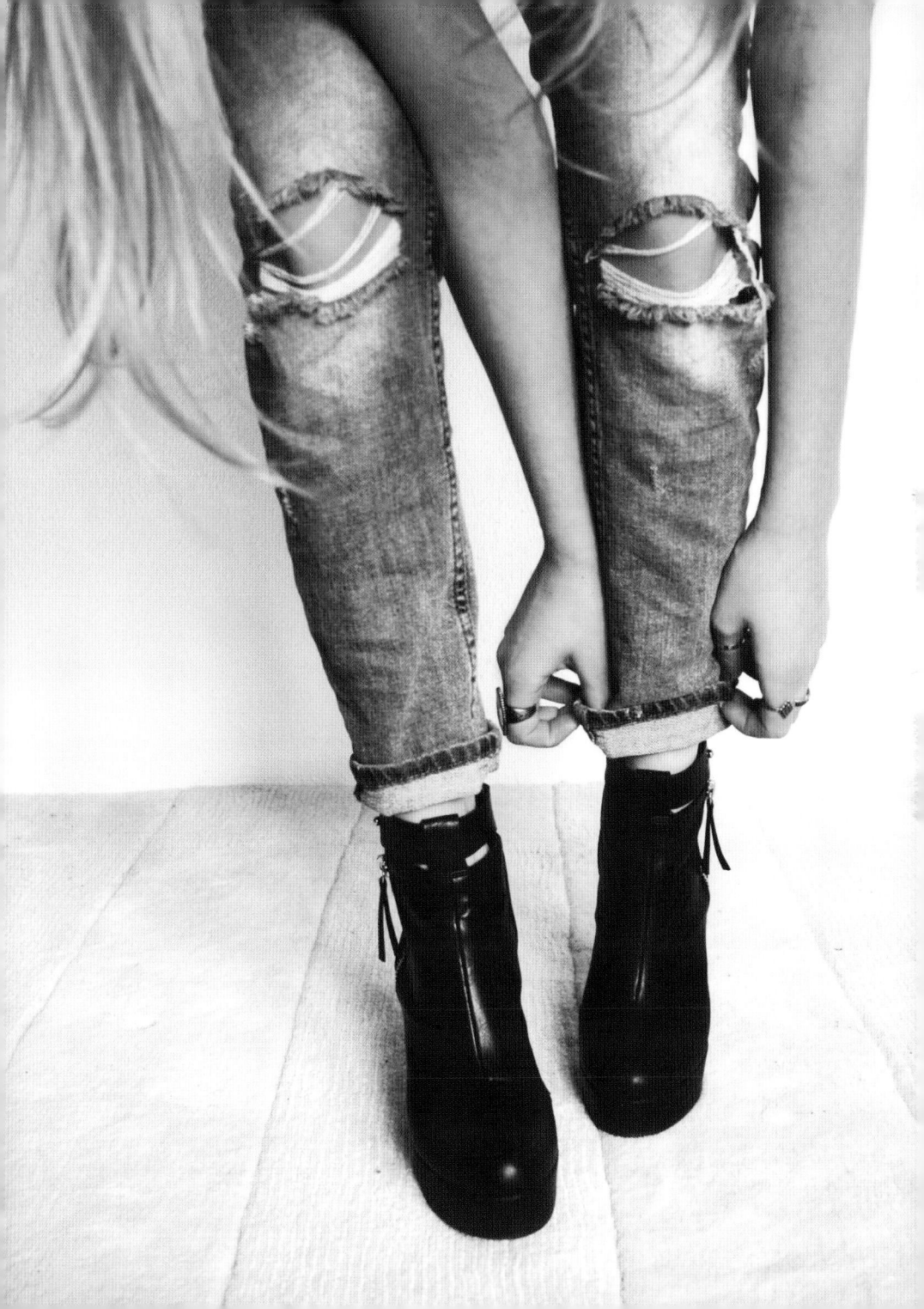

SHOES

WOMEN HAVE ALWAYS KNOWN

THAT THEY LOOK
BETTER IN HIGH HEELS

A great heel can change the shape and line of your leg muscles, making your legs look shapelier, more toned, and very attractive. The right shoe is the essential finishing touch to creating a perfect outfit.

Shoes should blend with your outfit through color, tone, and shape. They should be in the same color family as your outfit, but don't necessarily have to be an exact match. Your bag and shoes don't need to match either but they should be in similar style and proportion.

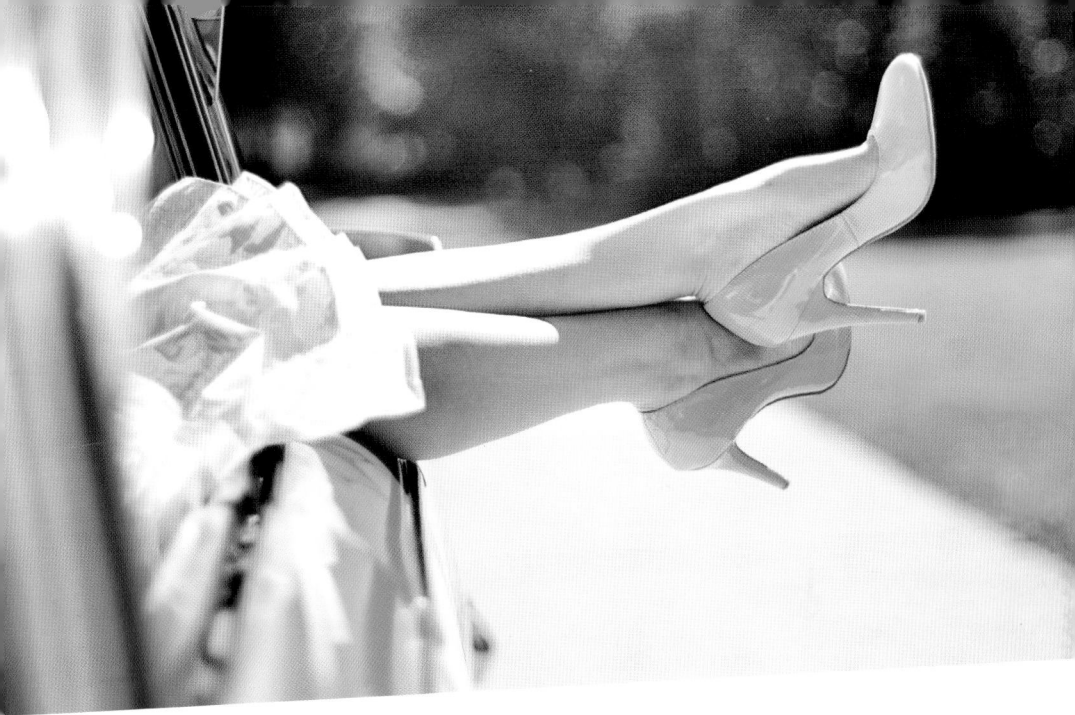

As a general rule, your shoes should be darker, not lighter, than your outfits (note the exceptions if you are going for a monochromatic look and want to use just one item to mix it up or if a fabulous nude pump makes your outfit pop). Black shoes may be too dark if you're wearing a very light or pastel outfit. There are other neutral colors (pewter, pale grey, and taupe) that will work better. Balance the weight of your outfit with your shoe style. If your ensemble is light and delicate, your shoes should follow suit. Thin straps, possible open toes, or strappy sandals with thin heels could all be options. Heavier fabrics like wool, tweeds, and corduroy need a sturdier shoe in order to offset the fabrics. Avoid bright white shoes; they'll make your feet look bigger. White pumps almost always look cheap, no matter how expensive they are. Try dark creams, taupes, and tan. Buy expensive shoes in neutral colors and classic styles so you can wear them for many seasons and they will go with most of your wardrobe. A slim heel will make you look taller and more elegant than a heavy, chunky heel.

Paul's Expert Tip

Heels can be great for a look, but sometimes you have a long journey or the weather is bad and you simply need to be practical. That is fine, but don't immediately revert back to your old running shoes which will just ruin your outfit. Get yourself one or two pairs of stylish sneakers, preferably in black or dark grey. They may not look as good as heels, but if you walk in the rain or need to take a train to the office, these can give you great comfort while still keeping your overall look intact.

No matter how fabulous those 5- or 6-inch heels are, make sure you can walk easily and with confidence in them and they don't throw your body out of alignment. When you have to spend a day or many hours in high heels, bring along another pair of heels with a lower height. It will keep you on your feet longer and you'll be much more comfortable.

When selecting which heel to wear, take into consideration whether you're wearing warm or cool tones. With cooler tones, wear shades of grey, pewter, and silver. Warmer colors need warm tones like various shades of bronze, copper, and gold. When buying metallic shoes, opt for the duller tones to draw the emphasis back to where it's supposed to be—your clothes and your face!

Black high heel pumps can be worn with almost anything and a good pair will last you a long time. Buy the best pair that you can afford, they should look expensive. Buy at least a 2-inch closed heel. Avoid very round, very square, or pointed toe shoes as your basics. A pair of nude or skin-toned pumps are another great basic. Ballerina flats are an invaluable choice for your wardrobe. Knee-high black boots, fitted to your calves, will take any outfit up a notch. Add some ankle boots and a more casual pair of boots.

Have you ever heard someone say that you should always eat before you go grocery shopping? Well, when you're shopping for shoes, try to venture out late in the day, when your feet are at their largest and sometimes slightly swollen from standing on them all day. Once you find the perfect pair that you just can't live without, try not to wear them two days in a row. I know it's going to be hard to resist. But the moisture from your perspiration will ruin your fabulous pumps. Check online to find a reputable cobbler in your area. Resole your favorite shoes as long as they're in good condition.

T-SHIRTS

A short note on this most misunderstood of clothing items. The humble T-shirt has become linked to oversized advertisements for sports teams and random meaningless slogans. Not that there isn't a place for those T-shirts, but people often miss the fact that these can be an easy, reliable, and inexpensive foundation for building your outfit.

A neutral T-shirt that is well-fitted and hangs nicely can be used with anything from jeans, pants, skirts, and shorts, it can be dressed up with a stylish necklace and blazer or dressed down with denim shorts and fashionable sneakers. It can even be used with a pantsuit instead of a blouse for work.

But the key is to follow my advice about all clothes: get the fit right, invest in good quality materials that hang well, and buy them in neutral tones (including white)—then you can wear them with literally anything.

ACCESSORIES

Now that you have built a solid foundation for your outfit, you can embellish things. The key to accessories is when in doubt, opt for simplicity. Choose simple quality pieces, considering scale and balance. Choose one perfect fabulous piece and that will serve you better than buying many cheaper, flashier pieces.

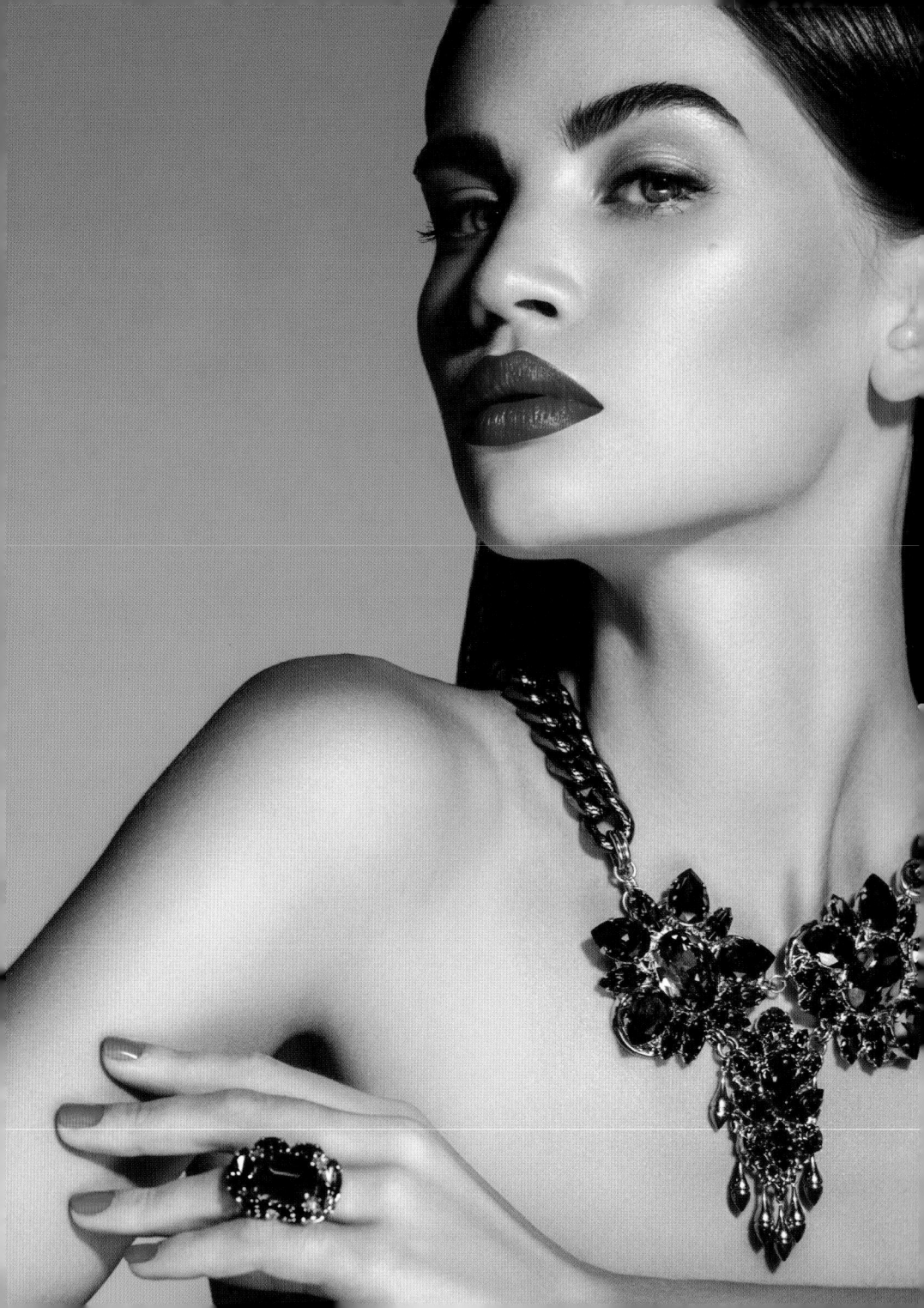

JEWELRY

When worn correctly, jewelry can frame and accentuate your features and elevate the most basic outfit. Take into consideration the size of your features, body type, and bone structure. These elements will determine the size of the jewelry that looks best on you. Earrings can brighten up your face and add sparkle to your eyes, making your face and neck slimmer. Experiment with different sizes of jewelry until you find the size and style that are most flattering.

If you're wearing one bold piece of jewelry, don't wear big prints. Instead, opt for solid colors, you will look much more chic. Wearing more than one piece of show-stopping jewelry typically doesn't work. Stick to a single unique or classic piece that makes a fashion statement. Try an embellished cuff or an elaborate necklace and if it looks great, stop there.

While simplicity is always safe, do not be afraid to mix interesting pieces together so long as they do not overpower each other. Mix classic jewelry with vintage pieces, and pricey, high quality gemstones with costume items. Try different accessory combinations to give each outfit added drama. Allow yourself enough time to accessorize and experiment with the finishing touches that each outfit requires. When wearing a lot of jewelry, group the items together instead of little pieces here and there.

The accessories that you spend the most money on should be classic pieces that can be worn from season to season. Invest in pieces that are more timeless than trendy. Pearls are always a good choice— they are classic, and flatter most skin types while they can be paired with evening wear, daytime dresses, or a fabulous pair of jeans.

SUNGLASSES

Let's be clear on this—the right sunglasses can make you look cool and are essential for the spring and summer or even a bright winter or fall day. They are a wonderful accessory that can work for any type of face or body, so take a little time to pick the right pair and you will enjoy them for years.

When choosing sunglasses, you want a shape that contrasts with the shape of your face. If you have a round face, look for square or rectangle-shaped frames. For a long face try horizontal frames. Experiment with different shapes until you find a pair that complements your face shape and then try different materials, such as metals, plastic, and lighter and darker frames that showcase your individuality.

There are many expensive and classic brands of sunglasses out there and those can last you a lifetime. But always remember to trust your own judgment; there is no point paying for a highly-priced designer pair unless they work for your face. If your budget is more limited, there are fantastic options in department stores, boutiques, and online in every style imaginable.

BELTS

My advice is always to replace belts that don't look stylish and top quality. Especially the ones that come with dresses and skirts (I know, I know, but it still happens!). They will usually look cheap and you can be so much more versatile and creative yourself. Remember, clothes should be fun so feel free to play with it.

Simple quality leather belts will always look great but this is an area where you can be bold if you have created a good foundation outfit. Jewelled or textured belts with statement buckles will work if that's your taste; try gold and silver chain belts, possibly a buckle with a designer logo (I've been adding flash to jeans and a T-shirt with my "H" for Hermes belts for years), soft, luxurious suede and rich crocodile and python skin belts are also desirable options.

PULLING IT ALL TOGETHER...

...FOR WORK

They say that in a job interview, the interviewer typically makes up their mind within the first thirty seconds. You may not be looking for a new job right now, but nevertheless the initial few seconds of meeting with someone is when those all-important first impressions are formed. Your style, clothes, and the way you wear them should represent the image you want the world to see. If your appearance is neat and well-organized, your co-workers and employers will assume that your work will be well-organized and professional. Whether it's a casual or more formal environment, always dress for the job you want. Let's face it, no one's ever been passed over for a promotion because they were too well-dressed.

That said, dressing for work doesn't have to be dull or boring. You can incorporate your personality into your wardrobe while keeping it polished. Start with a few key pieces and build four or five looks around them mixing textures and colors. Incorporate pieces that you already have in your wardrobe while keeping in mind the image you want to portray. Think of your work outfit as your brand.

The staples of your work wardrobe should be flexible and trend-proof—I will mention the stylish ladies on the subway in New York, London, and Paris once again, spilling out of the trains and heading to the office. They will have just a few simple, well-put together outfits and wear them over and over. It will save you time in the morning getting ready and ensure you are always confident in the workplace.

PULLING IT ALL TOGETHER FOR WORK:

III Dresses, whether shift, wrap, or sheath, should not be too fitted.

III Pants should have a flat front and be hemmed for heels.

III Skirts should fit well and not be too short, too long, or too tight.

III Pantsuits should be in neutral colors as well. You can add a pop of color with a top, blouse, or accessories.

III Single-breasted is best with a narrow lapel and pants that are slim cut because they are classic and trend-proof.

III If you can wear jeans to work, choose a dark rinse with a slim trouser cut that fits you well and remember my note on T-shirts—casual does not have to mean sloppy.

III Try carrying a structured tote with enough room for everything you need during the day, but don't junk it up! Totes are workday essentials but if you're messy, it will show to everyone who passes you at work.

III Keep it simple when it comes to the office. Pair basic styles with a cardigan or stylish jacket to complete your workday look.

III Do not, I repeat, do not wear tube tops, cut off sweats, or anything with a jagged bottom, flip flops, baseball hats, clothes that are too tight, skirts or tops that are too short, anything see-through or sneakers, or show too much cleavage. Also forget about sequins, Uggs, and message tees—these rules should apply even on dress down days!

Finally, make sure that you feel comfortable in your work wardrobe, as you will wear these clothes probably more than any other outfit.

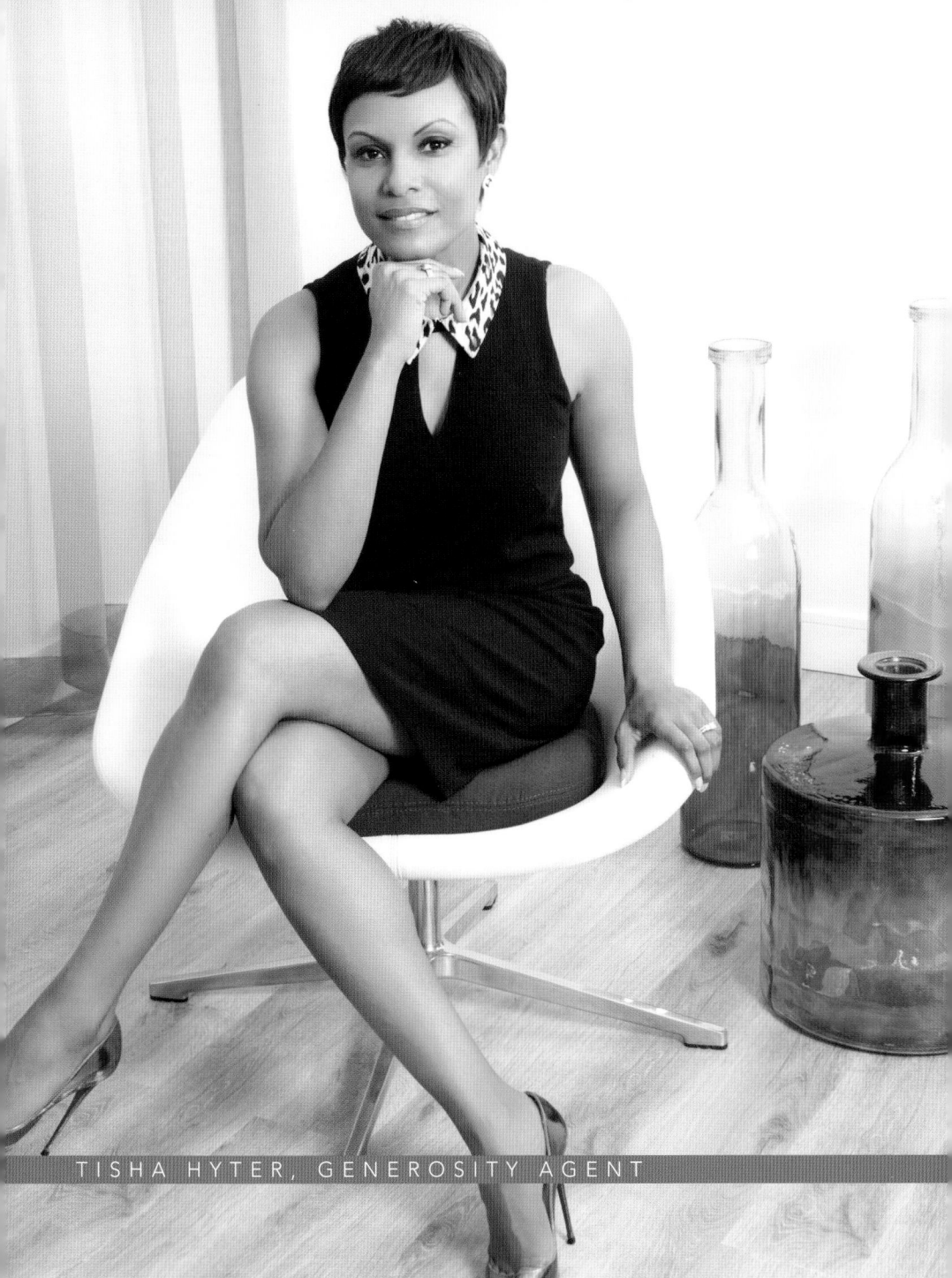
TISHA HYTER, GENEROSITY AGENT

...FOR GLAMOUR

Anyone who knows me understands that I love to get dressed up and hit the town. I hope that this book will help you feel more confident staying ready so you don't have to spend time worrying about getting ready. Getting glammed up should be fun, but sometimes the pressure of looking your best can chip away at the fun. I have a lot of ladies ask me about this and you'd be surprised how many women get nervous and can even have a great night ruined because they feel bad about their clothes and overall look.

Part of the problem is our expectation. Earlier in the book, I talked about us seeing images of stars arriving at awards shows and lavish red carpet events looking flawless, without a hair out of place, gowns perfectly stitched around

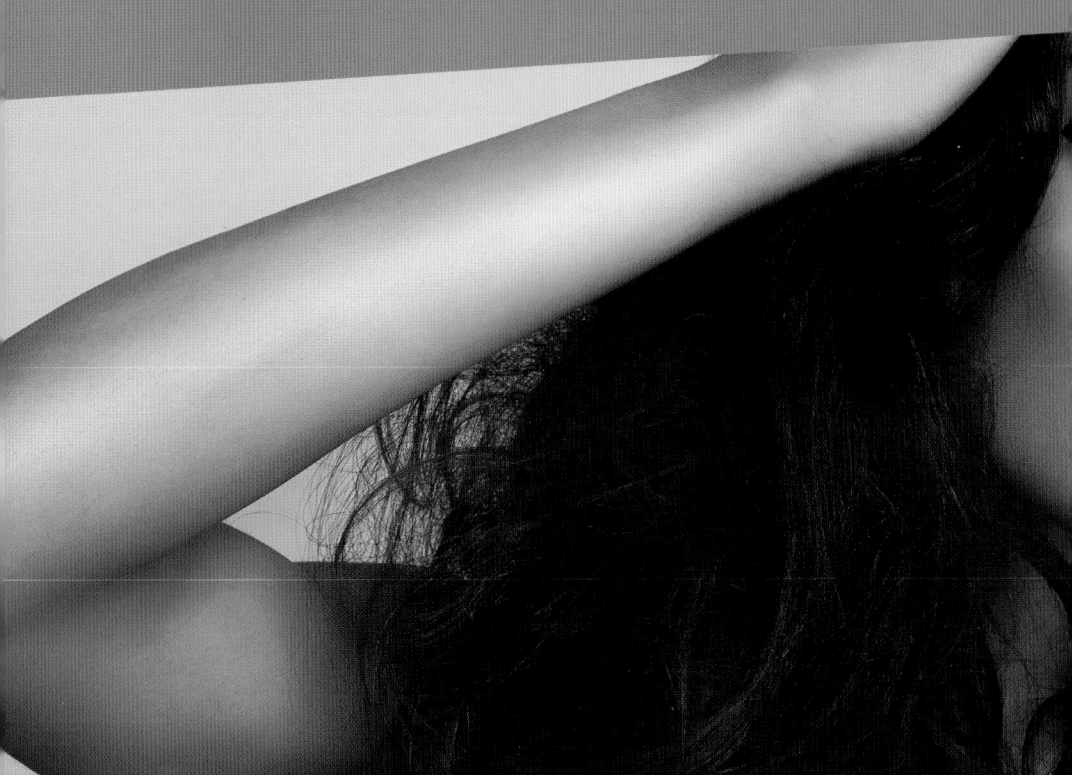

them, and dripping in obnoxiously expensive jewelry. Please don't forget that in most cases they've been assisted by their full glam squad which consist of a makeup artist, hair stylist, and wardrobe stylist. Most of the time, they'll have a stylist waiting just off camera to give them a touch up before hitting the red carpet. Also, they don't look like that all night long. Honestly, no one who has real fun on a night out looks that well put together the whole time.

That doesn't mean you shouldn't bring it when getting ready for a night out on the town—quite the opposite, but when you're getting ready, take the pressure off yourself, relax, and enjoy it. Getting ready should be part of the fun and the better you feel about yourself, the better you're going to look.

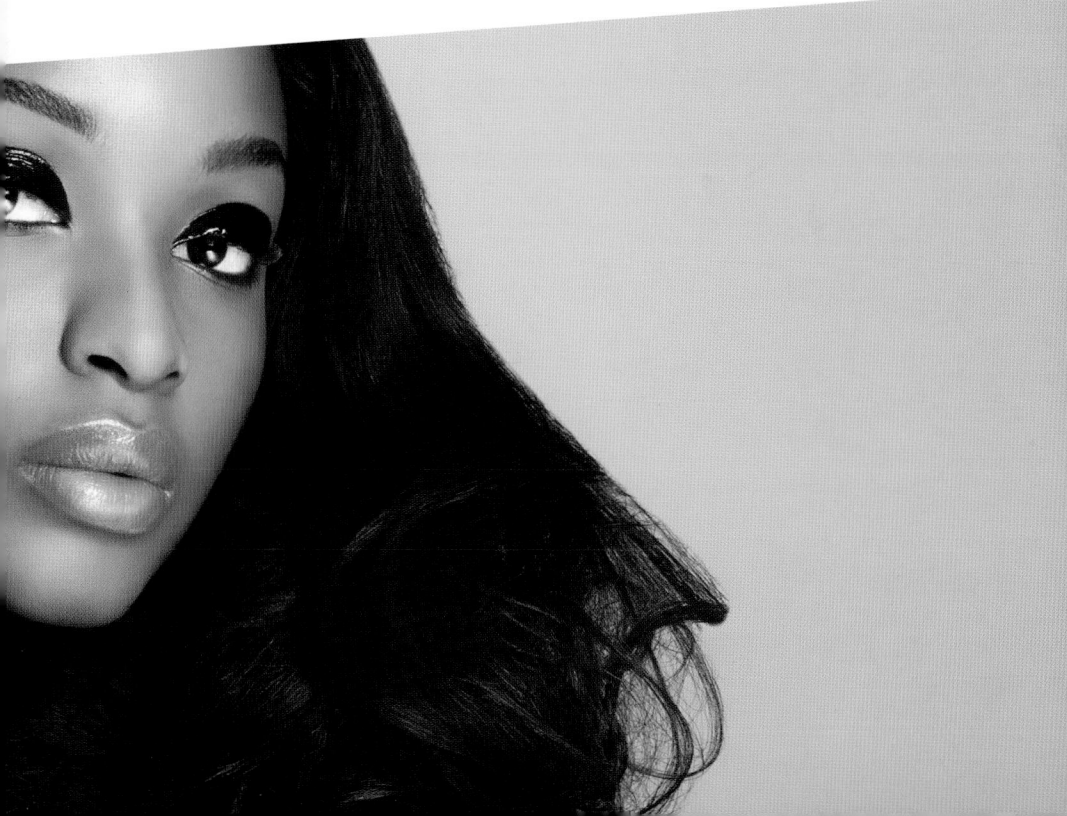

HERE'S MY ADVICE:

||| Firstly, follow all the steps I set out previously regarding fit and style. Dress for who you are—some ladies spend a fortune on designer dresses because they looked great on someone in a fashion magazine. Make sure the clothes you buy work for you.

||| Have a safe choice in your closet, and safe doesn't mean dull, it means "classic." For a lot of women, this will be the time-honored little black dress. You cannot go wrong with this—my advice is to try lots of different dresses in different stores and seek out a cocktail-style dress which comes down somewhere between your lower thigh and mid-calf. This is a versatile item that is worth investing time and money into—you can wear it without any extras as an understated classic choice or accessorize the heaven out of it and make it fabulous. Just think, what would your gay best friend do? Let that be your guide!

||| Know the event—always check the details of the party or event before you pick your outfit, remember you want to be glamorous but also comfortable so you can have fun and let go. For example, if it's a wedding, check if it's going to be outdoors or indoors, what the weather's like, will there be dancing, and so on. If you're going to a bar or club, think about the environment, is it a quiet and classy place, or a packed, sweaty party? Dress in a way that won't just look great in the mirror at home, think about how it will look wherever you are heading.

||| Less is often more—I get it, you have all these beautiful clothes, new shoes, fancy accessories, and jewelry that you never get to wear in the daytime, so you want to break them all out. But be careful not to overdo it; a few of the right items can make an outfit look incredible (see my tips on accessorizing), but too many of the right items can make you look overdone and sometimes junky. The outfit should showcase you, not the other way around.

||| Rock that clutch—treat your handbag on a night out as part of your outfit, it's another critical accessory. You shouldn't need lots of things when you go out: a credit card, some cash, a few portable makeup items, car keys or a subway card, and your cell phone. That's not to say your bag has to be small. The oversized clutch can look amazing, but don't clutter it with things you don't need. Remember this! We've all lost things when we're out so the less you take, the less you can lose. Keep your bag light and hold its shape, it's an extension of your outfit so choose it just like you choose jewelry. And never forget—have fun! This is your chance to let loose and enjoy fashion. All of my rules are guidelines and advice, but if you find a look that works for you that's not in my book, go for it! Having style is about finding what works for you. If you love it, it's in style and will usually look amazing out on the town!

...FOR EVERYDAY

I put this after the "Work" and "Glamour" sections for a reason. I wanted you to read all the other advice first and then finish here. I'm not going to go over everything again (you already know it now), but I really want you to take the pressure out of getting dressed in the mornings. When you're out running errands, picking the kids up, heading out to the movies, meeting someone for a quick, casual dinner, or whatever other regular activity you do, don't just go for the same baggy pants and T-shirt combo. You can dress well with little effort.

Follow the steps I set out by organizing your closet, building the capsule wardrobe, choosing only clothes that fit perfectly and work for you—once you have that down, every time you get dressed, it will look good because you have nothing bad in your closet. And the beauty of this approach is that you can get ready faster, meaning you don't need to reach for your old sweatpants and a baseball cap (nothing wrong if that's the look you want at the time, but it shouldn't be a default just because it's easy). Instead you can experiment more, trying out some different things, matching pieces together that you wouldn't normally try.

A FEW SIMPLE TWISTS ON CLASSIC COMBINATIONS:

⫶ Well-fitted jeans and a T-shirt can look great—but try adding a pair of ankle boots or statement shoes in a contrasting color to kick up the wow factor of the outfit.

⫶ A loose-fitting dress that sits around your mid-thigh to knee level can be worn by itself, or in the colder weather pair it with jeans or leggings and pumps. Add a belt for some structure, and you have multiple stylish but practical ways to wear that look.

⫶ Have a transitional jacket in your closet for spring, fall, and cooler summer nights—keep it neutral and in a classic style like a raincoat, an A-line, or even a simple biker jacket. That will go with almost any outfit and allow you to effortlessly navigate those strange days where the weather jumps between gray and rainy to bright and sunny in a matter of hours.

⫶ Don't be afraid to accessorize here as well, something as simple and useful as a classic watch can up your style game. You want to keep it simple because wasting time trying to match bracelets when you're late for an errand is never fun, but try out a few things when you can. Jewelry and belts have been covered, but if you feel adventurous then get a slim necktie and wear it loosely with a blouse or shirt, try some patterned scarves, and remember in the winter that a great a pair of leather gloves can make any outfit classier.

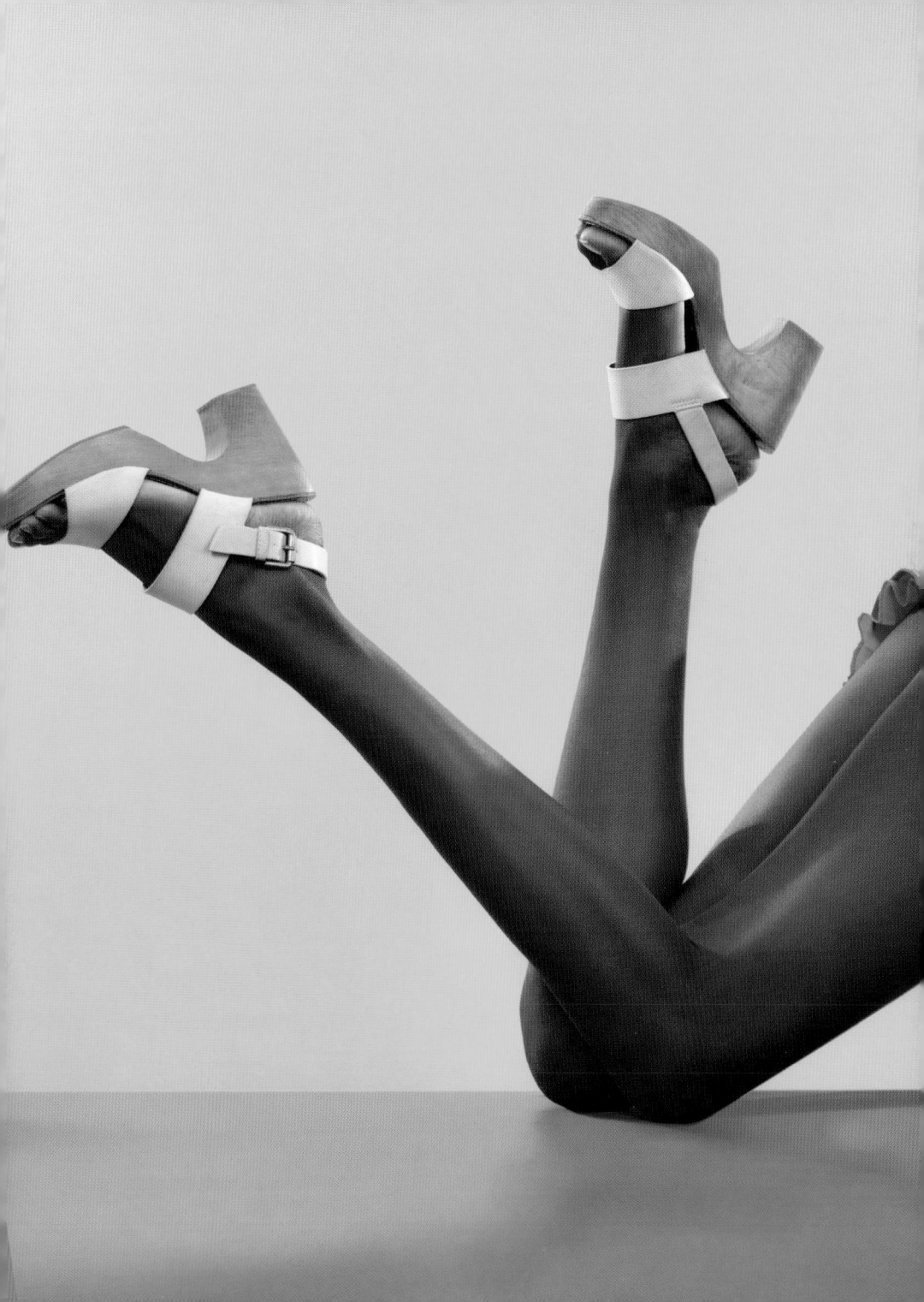

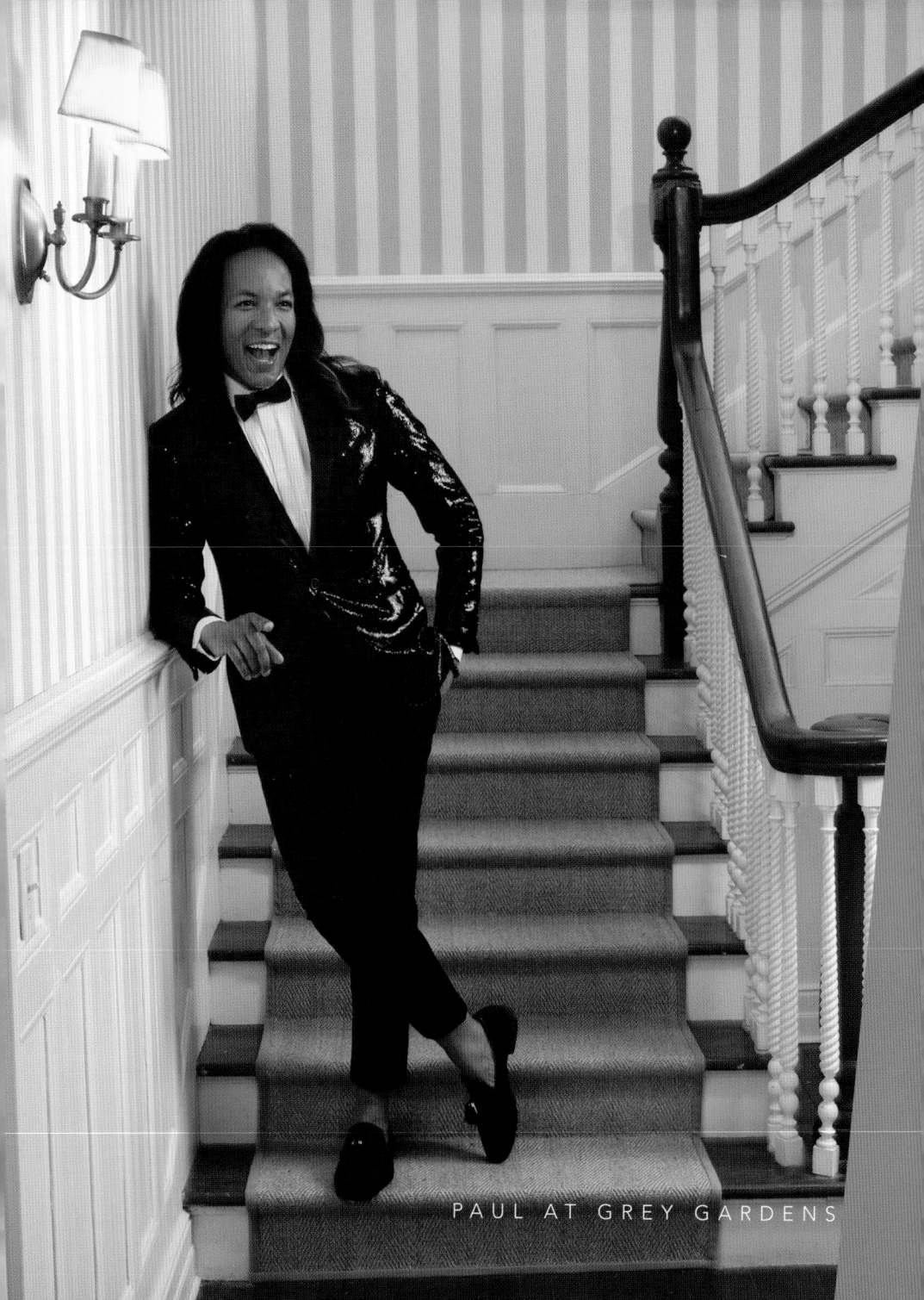

PAUL AT GREY GARDENS

PAUL'S LAST WORD

I want you to wear and enjoy all of your clothes! Fashion should be fun and make you feel good about yourself. Don't save fabulous pieces just for special occasions—enjoy them now. Shop for quality, not quantity, and try not to be an impulse shopper. You'll be overloaded with unwearable items that don't go with anything. Remember, keep it simple, focus on fit, comfort, and . . .

BE TRUE
TO YOUR OWN
STYLE

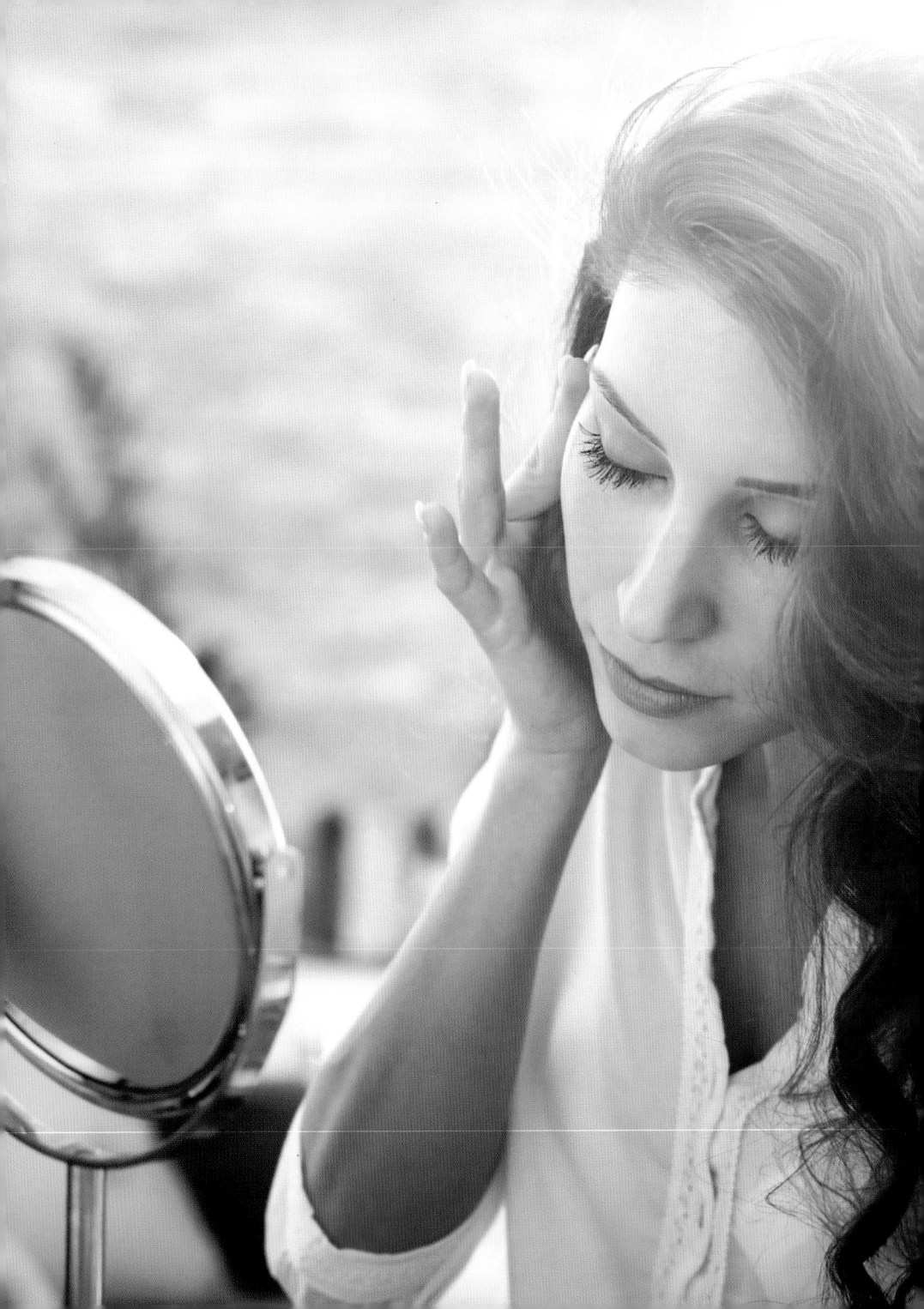

CHAPTER 2

ENHANCING YOUR NATURAL BEAUTY

HAIR & MAKEUP

HOW TO USE A MIRROR

I know, I know, you've been using mirrors your whole life and obviously you don't need me to tell you how they work. But I want to focus on how we process what we see staring back at us.

When I ask women whether they truly like what they see in the mirror, the honest answer usually breaks my heart, because they nearly always would like to change things about their looks. It seems most people classify the things that make them different as faults, instead of considering those unique traits attributes and unique signs of beauty. I'm going to start with this simple statement:

YOU ARE
PERFECT
AND YOU ARE BEAUTIFUL.

I know it's easy for me to say that and I don't even know you, but trust me, it's true. Forget what TV, magazines, and other media tell you is the right way to look or to be, I want you to remember at all times that there is no one definition of beauty, no single way to be.

So when you look in the mirror, I want you to try something (and I do understand how hard this is)—instead of immediately spotting things you don't like, focus first on the fact that you look amazing even before you've done anything and try to appreciate the features that you do like first.

I also want you to know that I'm not giving you makeup advice so that you can cover up your face and try to look like someone else. Just like clothes, makeup should be a way to dress yourself for different occasions, it should be fun, it should make you feel better. But you should never feel like you need it. Because you don't.

So, remember to use the mirror in the right way and if you don't feel like putting on makeup one day or don't have time, that's okay. You look amazing already.

BUILDING THE BASE–FOUNDATION AND CONCEALER

Just like most of the chapters in here, I could write an entire book on makeup and it would be divided by skin tone, age, skin type, etc., and there are many extra steps that could be added. But you're not here to become an expert on one thing; you want to know how to pull it all together, and that means understanding the basics and applying them to yourself in a time-efficient way that you can do with confidence.

Think of this as a simple guide to foundation and concealer. While many of you may know this already, you'd be surprised how many women I've met and coached who don't know why we use these or how to use them properly. Like so many things in life, you get shown one way by whoever was around at the time and you just stick with that.

I've separated this chapter a little and started with some real basics on both foundation and concealer as a kind of quick guide for anyone who needs a crash course. Afterwards, I break each one down into more detail and go over the key steps again.

WHY?

Foundation is literally that–the foundation of your look. Everybody's skin will be a little uneven with blemishes, slight tonal differences, etc. These are the wonderful things that give your face character. But when you're applying makeup to achieve a certain look, you want to set a uniform base layer so that you can build onto it.

But remember, you're not trying to hide your face or lose that character. Don't overdo it. Concealer also does what it says–it can help to cover up small blemishes (or big ones, depending on the type you choose) and it helps to create that uniform base of color that you can set everything on.

There are three very basic things to look at when you choose foundation: (1) color, (2) undertone, and (3) finish.

1 Always use a color that closely matches your natural skin tone (very important as I explain below in "Foundation").

2 Undertones are Cool, Neutral, or Warm—here is an old trick which is now popular online: without makeup on, stand in clear daylight and hold gold jewelry under your chin, if this makes your skin sparkle, you have a "Warm" undertone. If not, try holding silvery jewelry under your chin, if this makes you look good then you have a "Cool" undertone. If both work or you are unsure then you're probably "Neutral."

3 Finish is usually matte, semi-matte, or illuminating—matte is generally good for oily skin (but be careful not to over-apply), semi-matte will work for most people (so if in doubt, go for this), and illuminating increases shine to try and reduce the appearance of wrinkles (not for oily skin). Today's foundations can also be purchased in sheer, medium, or full coverage.

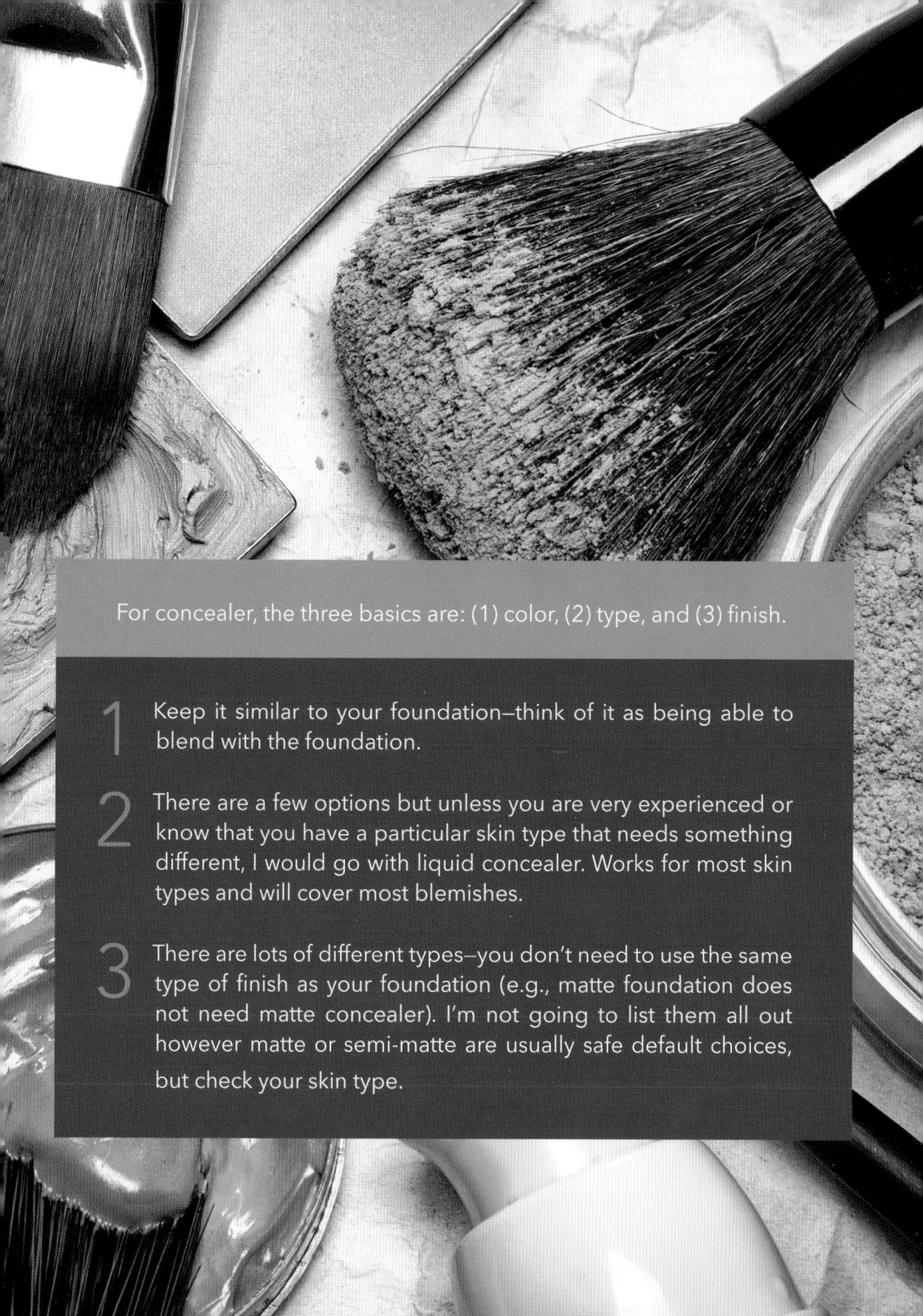

For concealer, the three basics are: (1) color, (2) type, and (3) finish.

1   Keep it similar to your foundation—think of it as being able to blend with the foundation.

2   There are a few options but unless you are very experienced or know that you have a particular skin type that needs something different, I would go with liquid concealer. Works for most skin types and will cover most blemishes.

3   There are lots of different types—you don't need to use the same type of finish as your foundation (e.g., matte foundation does not need matte concealer). I'm not going to list them all out however matte or semi-matte are usually safe default choices, but check your skin type.

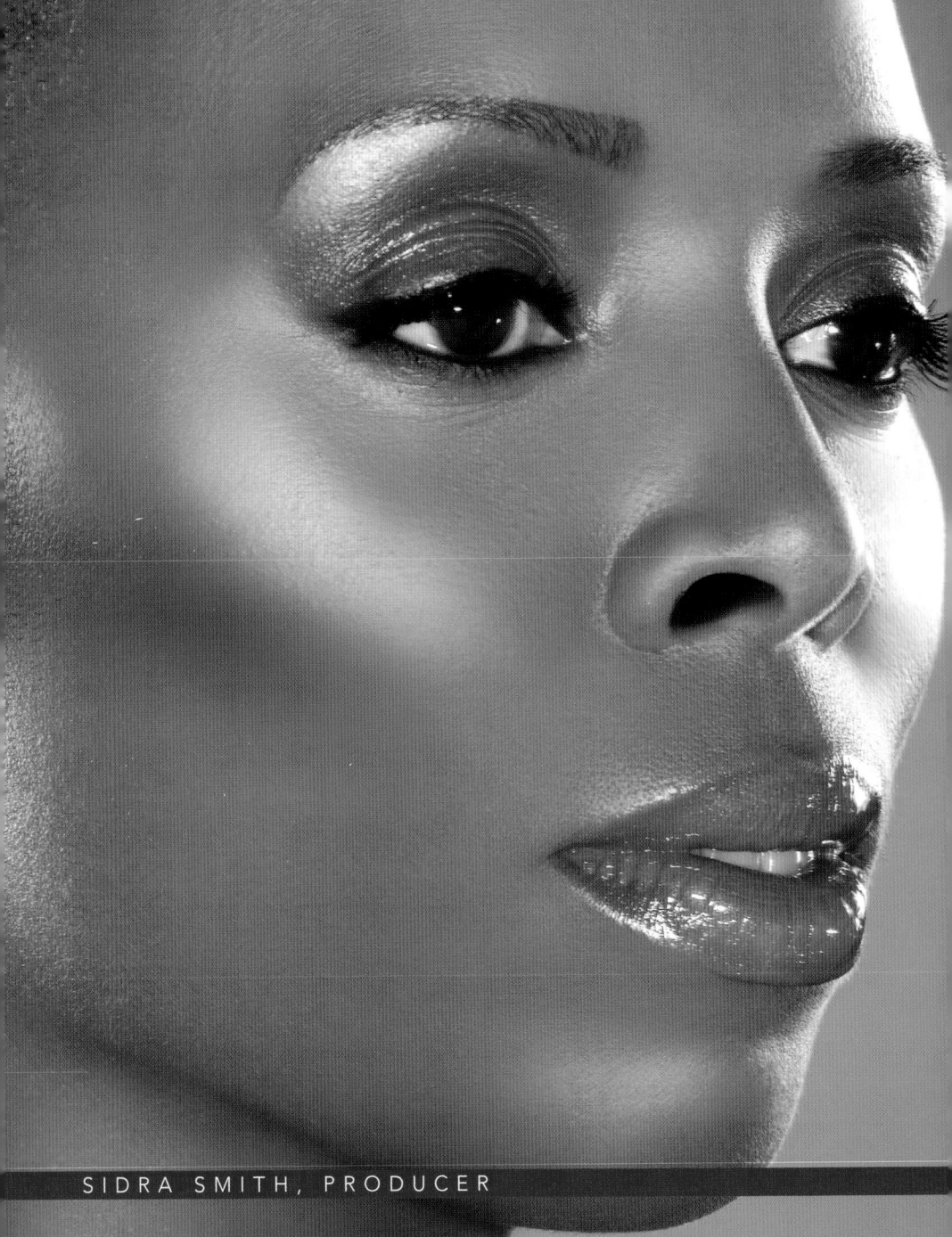

HOW?

Firstly, follow the steps in the next chapter on cleansing and moisturizing, do this before applying any makeup. Secondly, you can make the application as simple or complex as you like—I'm keeping it simple here.

- Start with the foundation (don't start with concealer, it will just rub off)—apply it across your whole face, I recommend broad strokes and make sure to blend it in so that it looks even across your skin. Start with less; it's easier to add more if you need to than to take some off if you go too far. You may not need as much as you probably think.

- Check your jawline, forehead, and by your ears—key areas where we often leave an imbalance or fail to blend properly.

- Concealer—I recommend just using a little bit on the areas where you see any particular blemishes or dark spots after the foundation has been applied. Again, less is more—if you dump a load of concealer, it will probably just look uneven and you're wasting an expensive product.

- Use a Kleenex to blot the concealer after you apply it, especially if you applied it near your eyes to cover up dark circles.

FOUNDATION

Now that we have the basics out of the way, let's really get into it.

Let's start with makeup primers. Most primers contain a silicone or similar ingredient that evens out any skin imperfections, filling in fine lines and large pores. They help your foundation and concealer glide on more easily. Prepping with primer before foundation will make your makeup go on smoother, more evenly, and last much longer. First, apply your moisturizer, then a primer if you need one. Your moisturizer needs to be applied first because it can't penetrate the silicone.

Primers, in my opinion, are best for sophisticated, more mature skin. The formulas that are silicone-based will fill in any fine lines and creases and enable your foundation to go on smoothly.

Foundations today are not just makeup; they're also skin care treatments. Some give a glow to skin with light-reflecting mineral particles that protect you from UV rays with sunscreen. They often contain antioxidants to fight off free radicals and some have wrinkle-reducing peptides and botanicals. Start with a light foundation; you can always add more if necessary, but if you think you need more wait another minute to give it a chance to blend in before you add again. Your goal is a moist, healthy look.

A word of advice: primer can be worn alone over moisturizer and a sunscreen. They help keep the moisture in and help balance out uneven skin tones, minimize redness and irritation, and help improve skin irregularities. If you want to minimize your routine or if you need to move quickly then this could be an option.

For a soft beauty (natural makeup) look, massage in a face serum for your skin type. It will smooth out your skin and help your makeup go on much more smoothly. You may only want to use a sheer layer of foundation lightly on your cheekbones, forehead, nose, and chin. Use a super light dusting of powder or none at all.

As I said before, never use a foundation that isn't a perfect color for you. The perfect shade of foundation should vanish into your skin without a trace and look like a second skin.

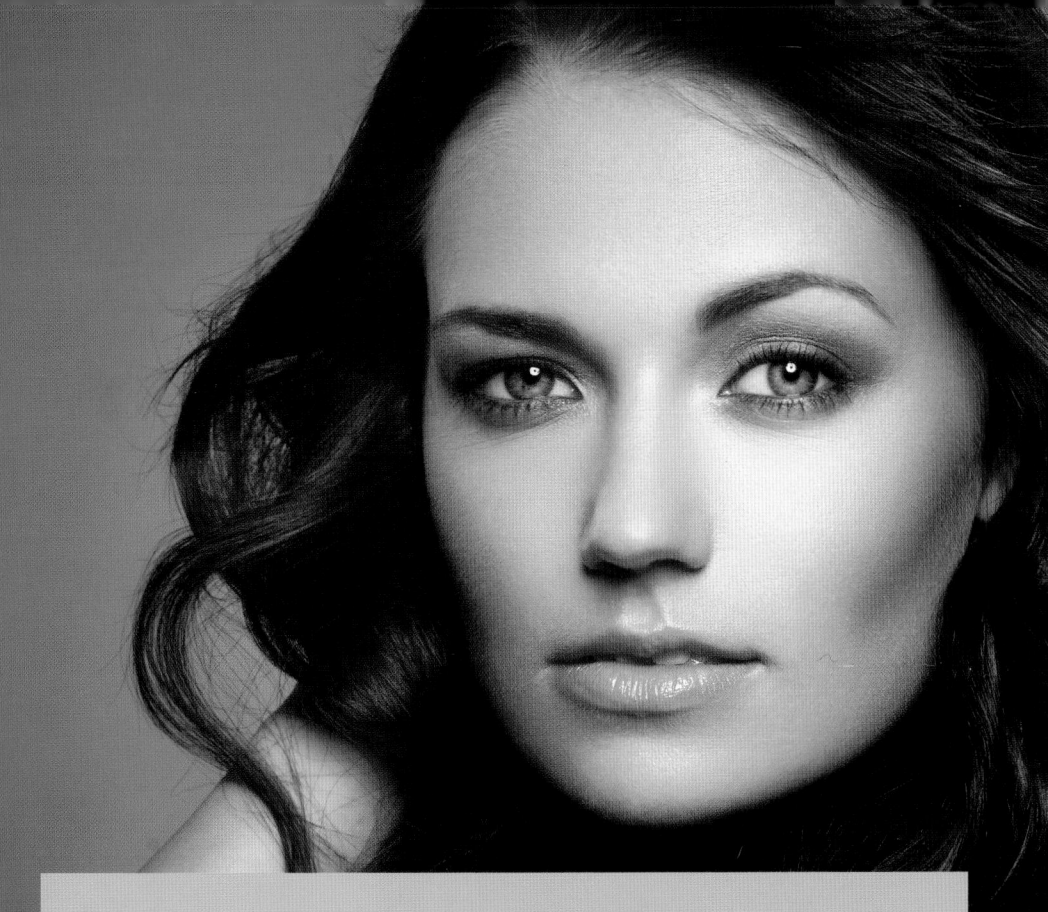

Paul's Expert Tip

Applying your makeup in layers will help it last longer and help you avoid using too much. Blend, and then blend more for a smooth, even complexion. Look for any streaks, smears, or areas that aren't well-blended. Make sure your skin texture is smooth before applying foundation. Foundation won't adhere properly to rough skin. Use a skin care regimen that works for your specific skin type.

Try some of the foundations that have light diffusers, moisturizing silk proteins, sunscreens from SPF 10–SPF 20, and even oil-free formulas with salicylic acid for blemish-prone skin. There are full-coverage formulas for covering age spots and uneven pigmentation that include antioxidants. Experiment with the different textures, they're sheer and lightweight, yet rich enough to give coverage and a flawless dewy complexion. Go with the lightest texture.

IT IS IDEAL TO APPLY YOUR MAKEUP IN NATURAL LIGHT.

If that's not possible, check out your makeup in front of a bright window before leaving the house to make sure everything's blended and looks natural.

Use your foundation to lightly even out your skin tone, not to cover, conceal, or hide anything. Start with the least amount of product, you can always add more if necessary.

Apply foundation, and then apply your concealer (more on that ahead). If you do this, you'll be able to see exactly where you still need coverage and exactly how much or how little you need.

You should always apply a sunscreen, even if your foundation has some sunscreen in the formulation. Usually there's not enough protection in the foundation and as you know, makeup moves around on your face and gets rubbed off altogether, leaving your face without protection. The sun is a wonderful thing but we need to protect our skin from it.

You'll need to re-evaluate your foundation color going from season to season. Your foundation in the summer can be a shade or two darker, since your summer skin tone tends to be a little darker than your winter skin.

When applying a powder foundation, make sure you've allowed enough time for your moisturizer to be absorbed thoroughly into the skin before applying your powder foundation. If you apply too much powder (foundation or translucent), dust a clean powder brush lightly over your face and it will remove some of the excess.

The goal with your foundation is to blend it well; if properly blended your makeup should be almost invisible and look like beautiful, natural skin. Any imperfections on your face should be concealed and blended with your concealer and foundation for a clear, clean canvas, ready for blush, eye makeup, and lips. Check your face in a bright light to see if all the colors and blending looks fresh and natural.

It's worth the money for women of color to buy high quality professional foundation. The ingredients in the higher quality products are better, especially products specifically formulated for black and brown skin. Lines like Fenty Beauty offer foundation in forty-plus shades, covering every hue from the lightest light to just about every shade of the deepest brown. Other lines are beginning to carry a wider variety of shades to ensure that all women can get a perfect foundation match.

CONCEALER

CONCEALER IS A MAKEUP ARTIST'S SECRET WEAPON.

Concealer is a makeup artist's secret weapon. They are formulated with concentrated pigment so a thin application will cover and conceal any impurities and undertones. They're smoother, more emollient, and lightweight, and conceal without looking greasy and heavy.

Almost all women need concealers. If you have clear, exceptional skin with only a few small imperfections, you may not need foundation. Choose a concealer shade that is the exact color of your skin and apply it only where you need it. Blend well.

Note: If you're using concealer, but not foundation, finish with a little loose translucent powder, to give your skin a more polished look.

Makeup artists recommend choosing a concealer that's one shade lighter than your natural skin tone. Stay close to the natural color of your skin, as cover-up that's too dark or too light will only accentuate your imperfections rather than conceal them. Yellow-based concealers are more natural on dark skin.

For women with oily skin, you'll want to find a creamy concealer that is non-oily. You want good coverage but you don't want clogged pores. First, gently apply a thin layer of your creamy concealer to any discolored or blemished areas of your face. If you need more coverage, add light layers until you have the coverage you need. Always blend well.

You should have at least two different concealers in your makeup kit. Buy a creamy, lighter concealer for under your eye and a more concentrated one for dark spots, redness, and other skin imperfections on your face.

Your concealer should have a rich, creamy consistency which is smooth to the touch. The concealer will spread more evenly and cover all your trouble spots. It should have a uniform color and blend easily. Many of the top makeup artists use two concealers for a seamless application.

When applying concealer that comes in a tube, scrape the tip of the wand applicator against the tube's rim to remove excess, then put several dots of concealer beneath each eye and gently blend. Repeat the process if you need more coverage. Blend well!

Word of advice: warm your concealer on the back of your hand first with your brush so it will spread more easily, since some concealers are fairly thick.

The texture of your under-eye skin is more delicate. If you find that your under-eye becomes easily irritated, mix your concealer with a little moisturizing eye cream.

For a more full-coverage look, use a stick or crayon concealer. They are creamier and more concentrated than liquid concealers.

If you apply too much concealer, add a small dab of moisturizing eye cream to the area and blend well.

There are certain colors that focus on specific trouble spots. For under-eye circles, use concealers with heavier coverage and light diffusing properties. The concentrated pigment in these concealers will also help cover veins and broken capillaries.

Do not use medicated concealers with acne fighters for healing and covering blemishes around your eye area. The skin around the eyes is very sensitive so treat it very delicately.

When using a light concealer under your eyes, don't apply it all the way to your lashes, it will make your eyes look smaller.

I always suggest applying an eye cream or gel to the under-eye area before using concealer. The concealer will go on much easier and last longer.

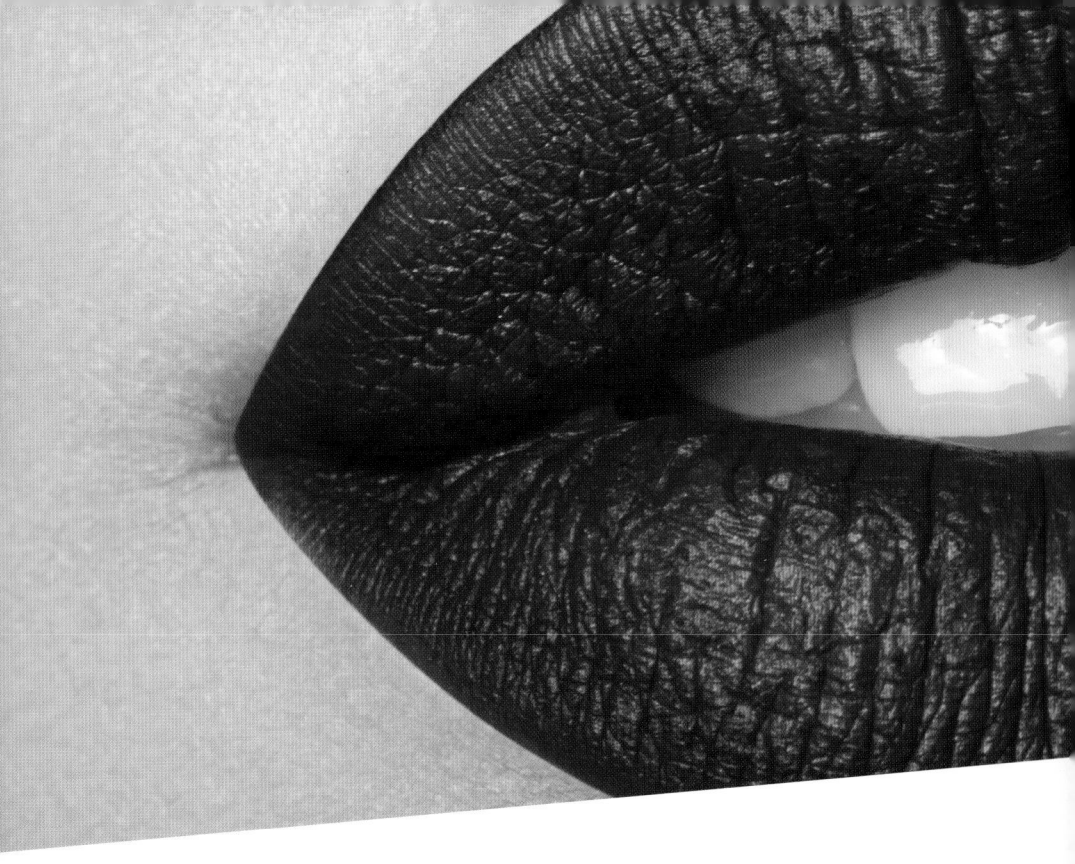

HOW TO POUT:
LIPS

Here is a failsafe way to apply your lipstick. Follow these steps and you will rarely find it on your teeth (don't you hate that?). Remember when you touch up or re-apply in the day don't rush, take an extra two minutes to do it in the mirror somewhere with space (i.e., not in your car while you're driving down the road).

1 MOISTURIZE—Apply a little lip balm, or even regular moisturizer in a pinch. Don't coat your lips heavily but just dab a little on in order to soften and protect.

2 CONCEALER/LINER—Some ladies swear by lip concealer and will always apply it next. Remember that you want to make this as easy as possible, the more steps you add the harder it is to stick to the system and you are more likely to rush. So, if lip concealer is your thing then go ahead—but if you've never tried it before, then I recommend going straight to the lip liner.

Use a liner that works with your lipstick shade (it doesn't have to be exactly the same, but find one that complements the color). Apply carefully starting from the outside in and following the outline of your lips doing both the top and bottom. Gently fill in the middle so that the liner covers all of your lips. This will hold the lipstick in place.

3 LIPSTICK—this is actually the simplest part if you prep properly. Start in the middle of each lip and work your way out. Always stay within the lips themselves and your lip liner (otherwise it won't hold at the edges).

4 BLOT—take a Kleenex, fold it in half, and place it between your lips. Then press them together on the tissue and open up again. Do not rub or pull at your lips, this blotting will help to take off just a little of the excess and make sure you don't rub onto your teeth.

5 CONCEALER—this is your facial concealer, take the product you just applied with your foundation and use a brush to work a small amount around the edge of the lips. Don't go over onto the lipstick, the idea here is just to define the lips and make sure the edge of the lip liner does not stand out. It is just like blending on other parts of your face.

As for the shade and color—I leave that to you to experiment, but that's the fun part, so do enjoy it and try some variations.

MY
EYES
ARE UP HERE

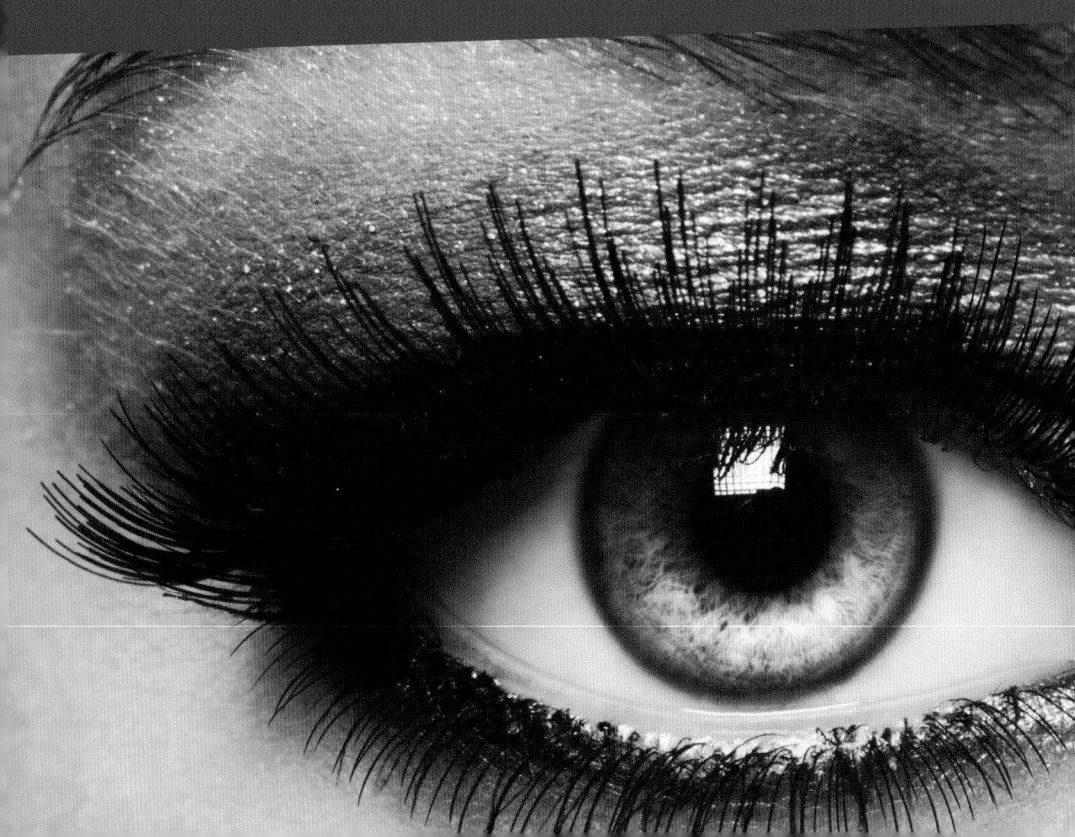

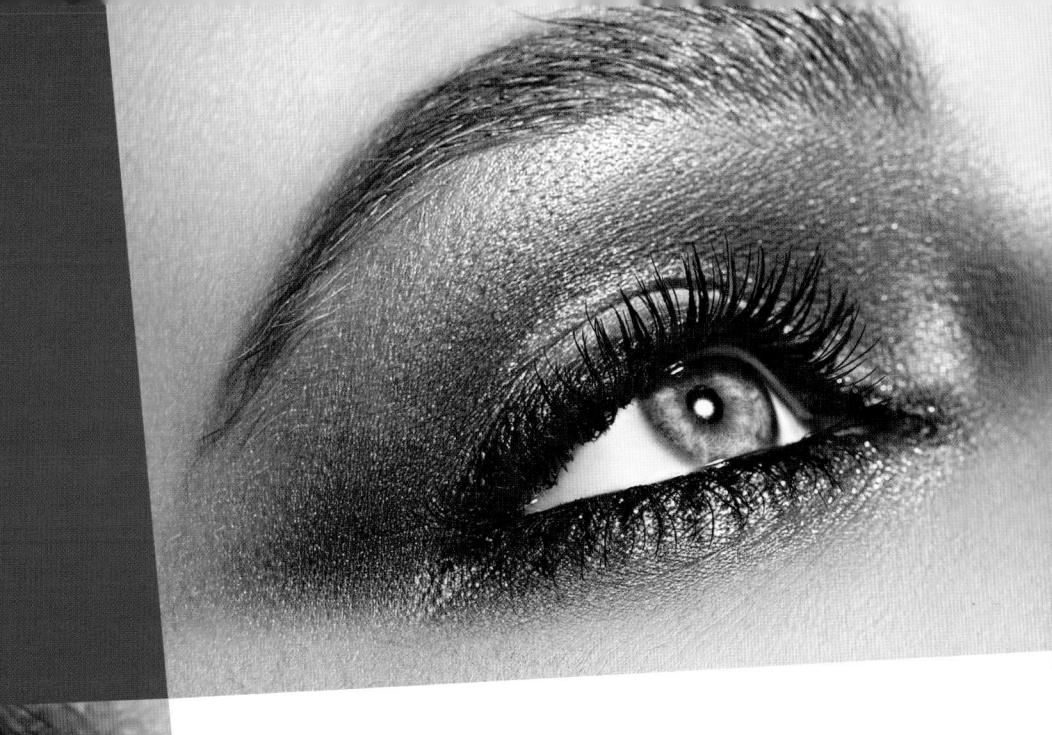

THEY SAY THE EYES ARE THE WINDOWS TO THE SOUL.

They are also one of the best features on any woman's face and you can make them stand out with just a few simple steps. Unlike the other sections, I'm not going to go through application of products—I'm going to be even more basic than that. This is because in my opinion the eyes, more than any other part of the face, are truly individual and you can make a bigger impact with them than anything else. It's also my opinion that women misunderstand their eyes more than any other part of the face.

I have set a few key areas that I think you should understand before picking up the brush.

EYEBROWS

Your eyebrows will set the structure for your face and your eyes. The great thing about eyebrows is that when done properly it looks totally natural and can lift your entire appearance.

This goes beyond tweezing between the eyebrows and trimming annoying hairs. You want to create a shape which includes the thickness of the brows and how high they sit. This is personal and depends on your face shape:

III Square face: Try a softer and rounded eyebrow shape but not too thin, you want to offset the strength of your jawline and soften some of the angles.

III Oval face: You don't want the brow to be too prominent; a gentle curve up and down in the middle of each brow will work with your face, but not too much.

III Long face: Take a flatter and more shallow line; you don't want to lengthen the appearance of the face.

III Round face: Be stronger with your curves; take the arch up a bit higher and don't cut it short at the end—you are helping to create extra shape in your face.

III Heart-shaped face: Keep it simple, don't go heavy on the angles, and just run a gentle curve up and down that follows your natural arch; less is more.

When applying makeup to your eyebrows you want them to look as natural as possible. Choose an eyebrow pencil in a shade that matches the natural color of your hair. Eye shadow in a shade that matches your hair can work double duty when

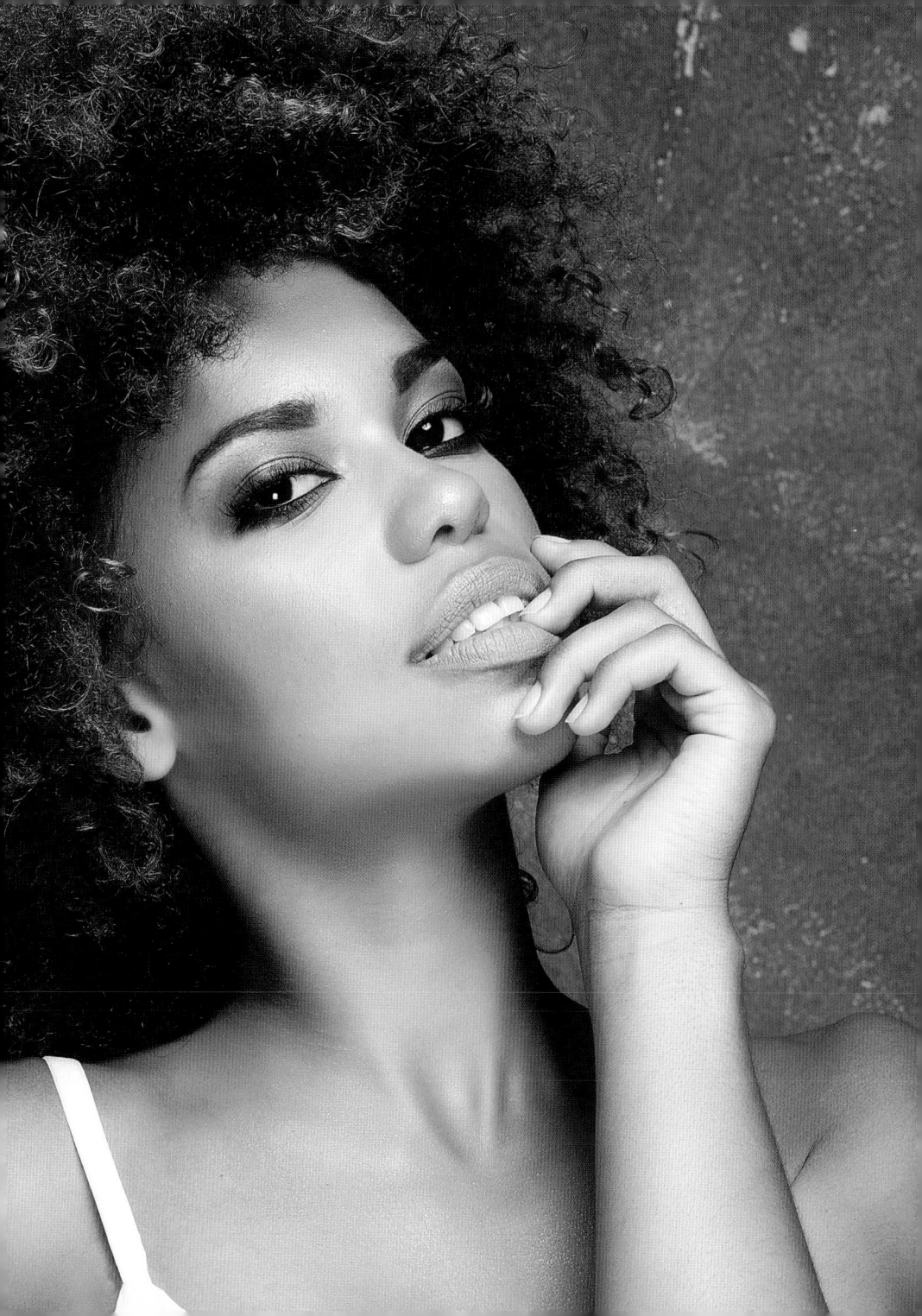

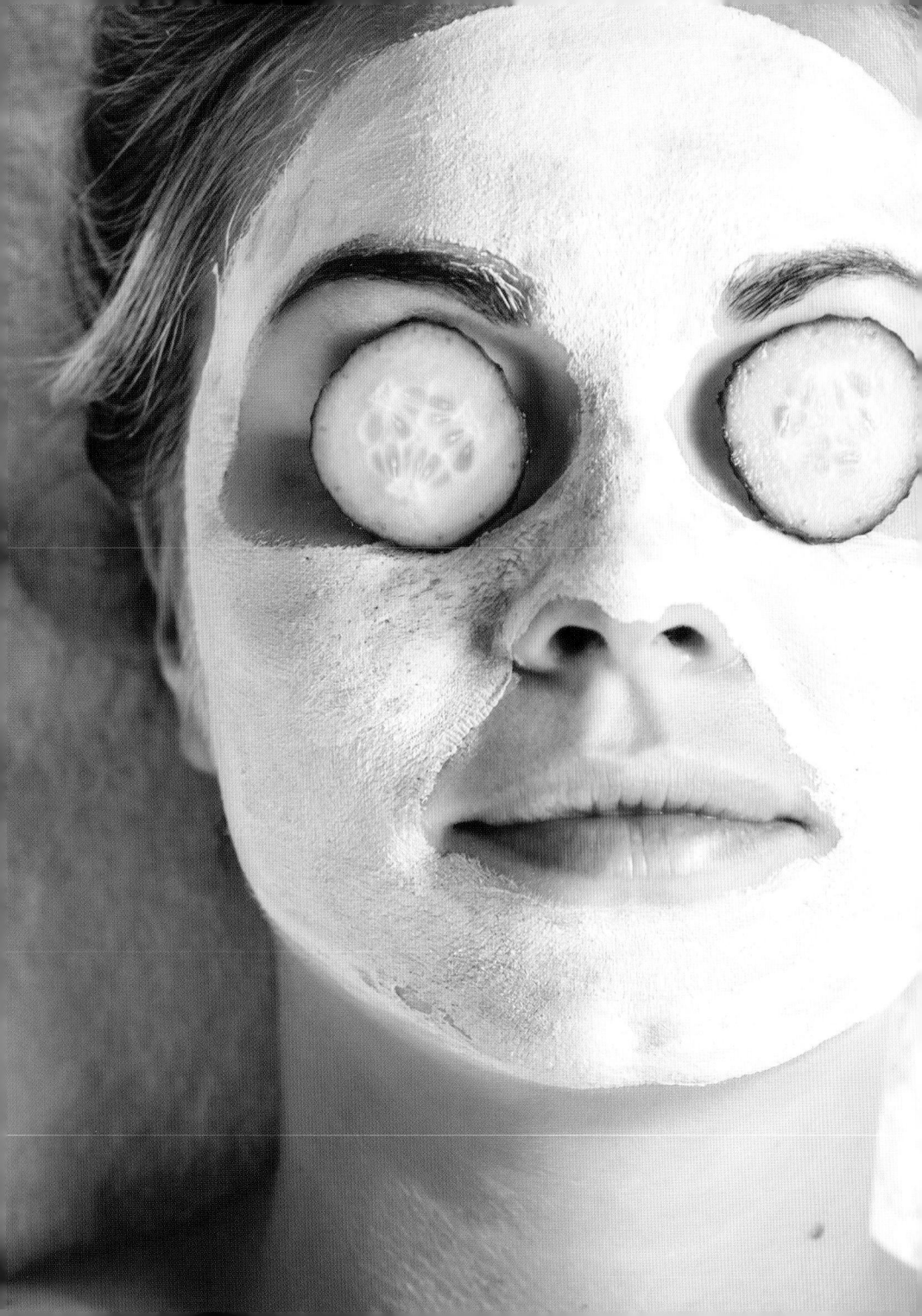

lightly applied to your eyebrows with a brush. Also, shades of taupe for brows are flattering on almost everyone.

Avoid drawing the dreaded solid, arched line to represent an eyebrow. This look is outdated and fake looking.

Fuller brows are fashionable now and more flattering and youthful for almost all women. This is one area where having your brows and arches professionally shaped is well worth the expense. Great-shaped brows frame your face and give you a polished look.

To fill in brows more naturally, use a brow pencil that's a little thicker than usual. It will give a thicker, less drawn-on effect. Apply a brow gel to finish the brow. Use a sharpened pencil for any area that needs filling.

HYDRATE

I realize you didn't expect to see this when dealing with your eyes, but one of the main reasons we use concealer around the eyes is to cover dark circles. Well, if you keep yourself well-hydrated (I mean water, cocktails don't count I'm afraid), it can reduce the existence of those circles in the first place.

COLD TEA BAGS AND CUCUMBER

Tea bags are an oldie but a goodie, take a couple of recently used cold teabags (they don't have to be chilled but it does help, so long as they stay moist), close your eyes and place them under your eyes first thing in the morning for at least a few minutes, but fifteen minutes if possible. This really helps to reduce puffiness in the eyes and makes you look fresher.

Cucumber has been around since the dawn of beauty regimes, but I'm including it because recently several of my clients have been questioning whether it's an old wives' tale. Well, it ain't–cucumber slices first thing in the morning on each eye really do help reduce dark circles.

Try to keep them on for at least fifteen minutes.

If you want to take a modern approach, use a de-puffing gel to drain excess water from lids each morning.

For a puffy face, try taking an aspirin. Aspirin has anti-inflammatory ingredients that will calm down a puffy face.

SLEEP

I've said it in several chapters of this book, sleep is like a magical thing that can fix all manner of problems. It will improve your eyes—if you can get your head down just an hour earlier each night, you will see the benefits in your eyes.

EYELINER

Liquid eyeliner is the most difficult makeup to apply. Try substituting the thin brush that comes with it for a flat tip synthetic brush that's a little wider. Always paint right along the root of the lash hairs for a thicker, foolproof line.

Use a flat or angled liner brush to apply your eyeliner and run it through one of the new gel liners, for a creamier, liquid texture. Apply liner close to the lash line, filling in the spaces between your lashes as closely as possible. Sparse, thin lashes will look much fuller and lush. The line will look more natural and your eyes will stand out. The line should be thinner at the corners of your eyes and heavier in the middle to accentuate the roundness of your eyes and lightly line under the eye.

Try mixing cake eyeliner with a few drops of Visine and apply with an eyeliner brush for more staying power.

EYE SHADOW

Use your palest eye shadow shade as a base to neutralize the lid color and prime the eyes for a long-lasting crease-proof color. Use eye shadow to line, define, highlight and contour the eye. To prevent your eye shadow from creasing, prime your eyelid with concealer or foundation on the lids. Apply eye shadow, and dust with a translucent powder.

You can also use your eye shadow to line your eyes. It gives a softer, more natural-looking effect than pencil or liner. Use a thin, angled brush, pick up some of your shadow on it and dot it across the top of your lash line.

Natural nude and neutral is the new way to wear eye shadow. Browns are subtle and look good on all complexions. Depending on how they are applied, they can go from a natural daytime look to a smoky, sexy eye for the evening.

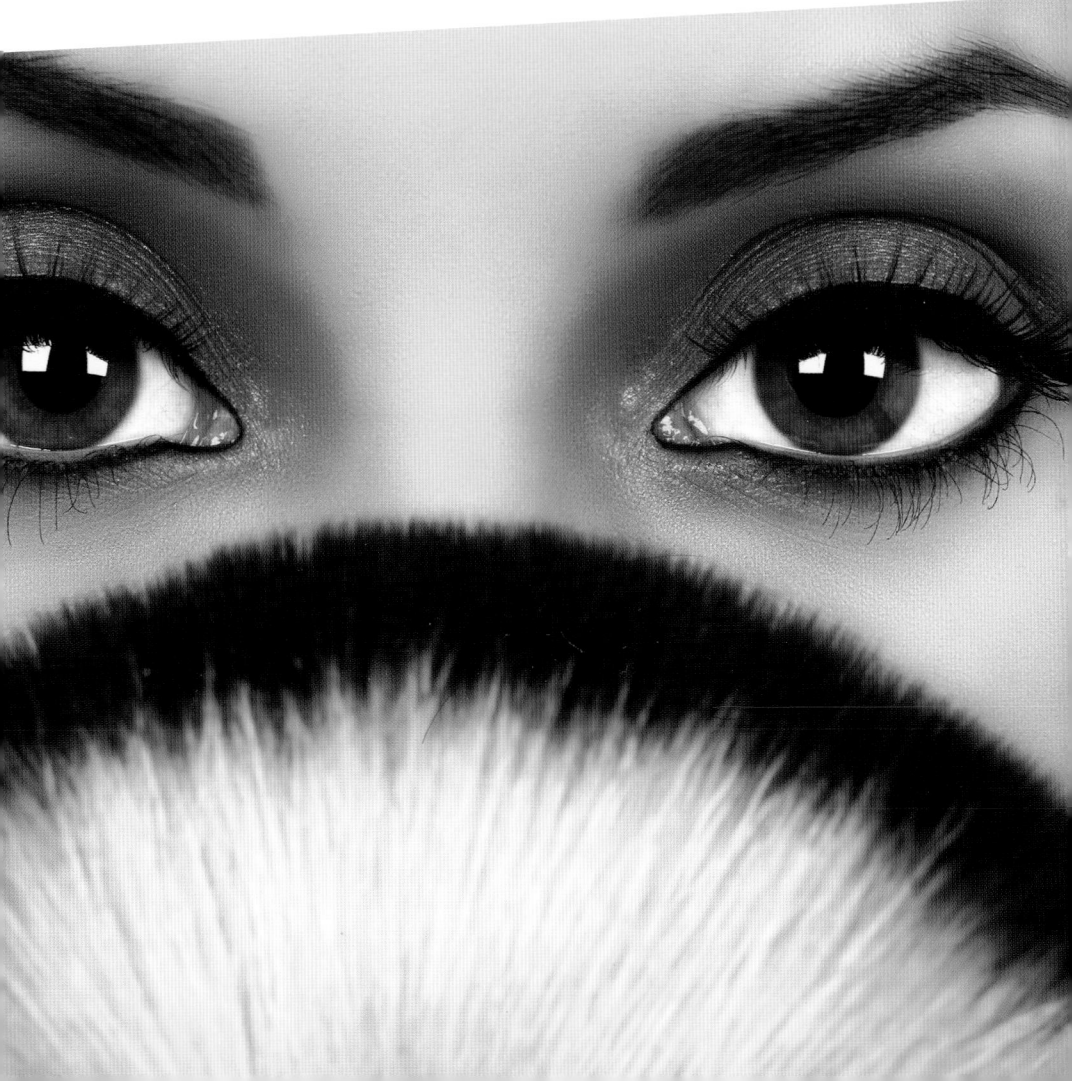

HERE ARE A FEW TIPS ON EYE SHADOW:

▮ If you have a fair complexion, choose browns with a hint of pink, muted, tawny earth tones, bronzes with a rosy tone, light, and dark colors. Start with a beige taupe base and add some shimmering golds and bronzes.

▮ If your complexion is medium, choose a shadow a few shades darker than your skin tone to give some balance to your look. Taupes and coffees, cappuccinos and toffees, will all heighten your look. For evening, layer some silvery pearly shades over your pale brown tones, or layer a golden cream shadow over a matte chocolate base.

Paul's Expert Tip

When applying makeup or eye treatments to the area around your eyes, bear in mind that the skin around the eyes has no sebaceous glands, making it drier, much thinner, and more delicate than other skin on your face. I keep repeating that because one of the most profound ways for us to look older is by neglecting the eye area. Also, there's no fat there for padding, so that area is more prone to puffiness. When applying eye creams, use a light touch. Lightly pat, then gently press and roll with your ring or pinky finger. Apply from the outer corner of the eye to the inner corner. Investing in a high quality eye cream with a rich gel-like texture is usually well worth the investment.

▮ Olive complexions have golden undertones, so use coffee, chocolates, bronzes, and butterscotches and mahogany. Use a sheer layer on top for a sultry, mysterious look. Use a dark brown pencil to line lids close to the lash line, and then smudge for a smoky look.

▮ Dark skin can throw caution to the wind and pull out the dramatic, intense colors. Avoid colors that are too brown—instead, choose rich coppers, bronzed chocolates, deep touch-ups. Try layering a dot of glitter eye shadow over your base eye shadow in sheer gold cream or iridescent bronzes.

DARK CIRCLES

To try and reduce circles, use a product that has vitamin K, retinol, or kinetin. These ingredients contain coagulation ingredients that help strengthen blood vessel walls, so veins become less visible. Lasers may be an option for very severe and constant dark circles.

Choose a non-cakey liquid concealer for best results. The darker the circles, the thicker the consistency of your concealer should be. You may be able to use a lighter consistency concealer, but just layer it. With light to medium dark circles, you may get enough coverage with a creamy semi-sheer concealer. Try one with light-reflective particles.

Use a loose translucent powder to set concealer; a pressed powder can sink into the fine lines and accentuate the problem areas.

The skin under your eyes is thinner than other areas, so the red and blue blood vessels tend to show through more readily. First, apply a quality eye cream or a rich moisturizer, since that area under your eyes lacks oil glands. Your concealer will be much easier to apply.

Cold compresses may also help with dark circles as they do with puffy eyes. They will help to temporarily shrink the blood vessels causing the darkness and may lighten up the area.

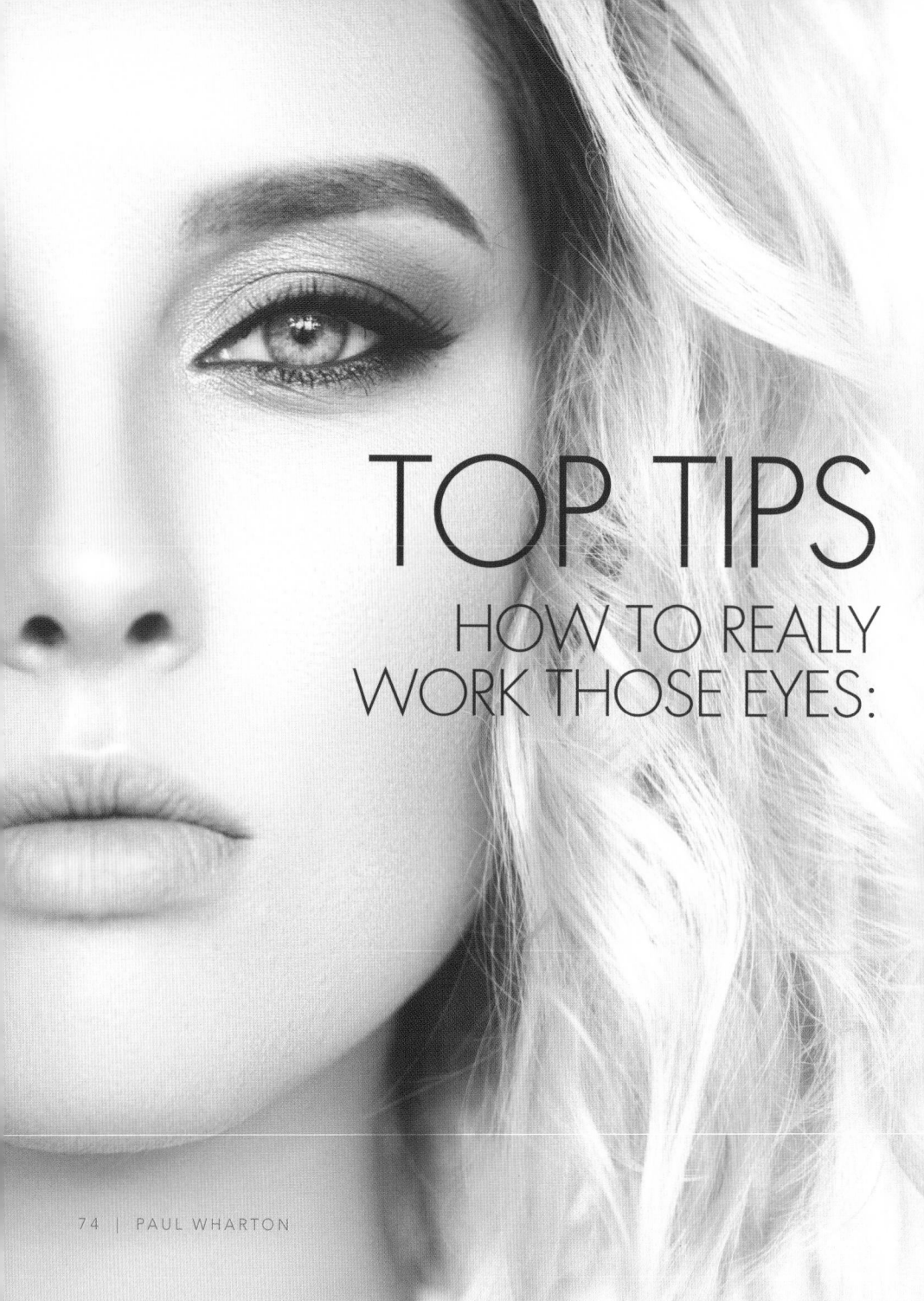

TOP TIPS

HOW TO REALLY WORK THOSE EYES:

III Lift and brighten your eyes by using an eyelash curler. It will instantly open up and accentuate your eyes. After curling, apply mascara to the top lashes.

III A sexy, smoky eye doesn't have to be black. The key to a smoky eye is a subtle smudging of the color around the rim of the eye. Dark grey, dark browns, and dark purples will work.

III The skin beneath the eyes contains less collagen and elasticity than the rest of the face. That means this area is the first place swollen blood vessels, excess fluid, or fine lines show up when you're tired.

III Dark circle treatments can cause skin sensitivity and temporary redness and are best used in the evening, as are anti-aging creams, because cell metabolism peaks then.

III For fine lines around the eyes, choose moisturizing creams with ingredients like hyaluronic acid, soy, and vitamin E. Apply a small amount under the eyes, then pat gently with your finger to blend. Repeat with a dab on your upper lid, smoothing up the brow bones. Wait two minutes to allow it to absorb into the skin.

III In warm, humid weather, eye makeup runs and creases. Try using a waterproof pencil to line your eyes. Then gently smudge.

III For longer, lush lashes, hold the mascara wand vertically and apply the mascara sideways, back and forth between the lashes. Comb through the lashes to evenly distribute the mascara from the base of the lash to the tip.

III To keep your mascara from clumping, use lengthening, not thickening, formulation. Only apply two coats and comb through to remove any excess product.

BLUSH, BRUSHES, TIRED FACE, TANNERS & EVERYTHING ELSE

I really wanted to talk to you about a few other aspects of makeup but I didn't think they all needed a full section, so I put them together here. We've covered the face pretty well, but I've included here a whole set of advice including your body, feet, and how to overcome that dreaded "tired face."

BLUSH

Blush can really set off a look, so why didn't I include it earlier? Because it's not essential and I'm trying to give you advice to help you be efficient. But, if you have time, definitely reach for this product.

The blush colors that generally look most natural on your face are soft shades, such as soft pink, rose, peach, subtle plums, and even tawny pinks. Colors that are too dark, too brown, or beige may look dull and muddy. Be careful not to use too much color or not enough, and I would say avoid frosts and shiners; they draw attention to any lines or flaws on your face.

- Fair skin looks best with pale pink and pale peach shades of blush.
- Medium skin can wear a wider range of colors: pinks with a little deeper color and tawny pinks.
- Dark skin needs more color. Blush colors should be deep enough to show up on dark skin; try plums, reds, rust, and vibrant raspberry.

Nothing flatters your face and bone structure like a little highlighter along your cheekbones and towards the temples. Also, a little highlighter under the brow bone looks great. Your whole face will look radiant.

For long-lasting blush, use a cream blush on the apples of your cheeks, set with a translucent powder. For extra staying power, add a dusting of powder blush or bronzing powder on top of that. When applying powder blush, always tap the brush to get rid of excess product.

If you apply too much blush, just apply some translucent powder over it to tone down the color.

Women of color should avoid blush that is too pink—yellow undertones, with peachy, tawny blushes will probably work best. If your skin is dark or very dark, rich cinnamons, plums, and deep berry colors will look great. Adding a bit of gold shimmer will lighten up your whole face and you will look spectacular. You can experiment with deep, rich colors that accentuate your beautiful skin color.

BRUSHES

The secret to natural, great looking makeup is proper blending. And the secret to well-blended makeup is professional quality makeup brushes.

Good makeup brushes (properly taken care of) will last a long time and be well worth the effort and cost. Don't try to buy them all at once. Buy one quality, well-shaped brush at a time. Medium and long length handles are best for application; the smaller handled brushes are of course more convenient for travel and to throw in your purse.

Good quality brushes can be found at an art supply or craft store. They come in all sizes and some are shaped perfectly for shading and eye shadows.

Make sure to care for your brushes. Clean them at least once a month with a brush cleanser, shampoo, or mild liquid soap, and occasionally an antibacterial soap. Use towels to press out water, then allow to air dry.

Sharpen eye and lip pencils frequently to remove bacteria. Other products can lose their effectiveness within months once they're opened. Discard any makeup that smells or looks strange.

TIRED FACE

Stayed up too late? Too much partying? We've all been there. Here are some tips to make you look more rested and hide the obvious signs of your fun (or work) the night before.

While cleansing, give your face a light massage to stimulate the blood flow. Use very little powder, if any at all, as it will make your face look more dull—unless it's a luminizing powder.

Sleep lines can be eliminated with a very warm washcloth held against the creases and lines in your face until it cools and the lines lessen. Dry your face with a hair dryer set on the cool setting. This will give your face a dewy, youthful glow before you apply your makeup.

To wake up tired eyes, try a bit of pale yellow eye shadow if that works with your skintone. Use on the brow bones or wherever your eyes tend to be red.

For dryness or redness in your eyes, always keep your eye drops handy. Use moisturizing eye drops to moisten and cut down the redness.

For more advice on reducing puffiness in the eyes, check out my chapter on skincare.

TANNERS

While I've got your attention and focus on makeup, I want to talk sunless tanning products. These can be great for just about every skin tone. The purpose is to make your skin glow and really enhance that canvas on which to apply your makeup. But you need to use them in the right way. I see too many women with poorly applied tanning products and it ruins their entire look. Also, if you're going to use sunless tanners, make sure you adapt your makeup choices—your skin tone will be different depending on the tanner and how long ago you applied it.

The secret to applying self-tanner is to first exfoliate skin in a lukewarm shower (see my tips on exfoliation in the skin care chapter). Apply a light, non-greasy moisturizer to your face and body, allowing several minutes for it to sink in. This gives you a clean, even area for application. Always use face tanners that are made specifically for the face. Formulations that are designed for the face usually won't clog your pores or cause breakouts.

For a longer lasting tan, always moisturize your skin after you've achieved your desired tan. If your skin is extra dry or dehydrated, apply a rich moisturizer after your self-tan has soaked into your skin and the tanning process is complete. Avoid using self-tanners before you work out, as the excessive sweating will cause it to streak. Wait a few hours to make sure your skin is completely dry.

Many dark-skinned women use sunless tanning products to give their skin a bronzy, coppery glow. A little added color helps to eliminate any shallow or ashy tones that occasionally appear in dark skin. Use dark and intense formulas for a darker tan. These products have the most active ingredients.

Note: If you want to use a bronzer you may need to apply blush first. Adding and blending bronzer to your blush gives a healthy sun kissed look. Add to areas where the sun would naturally hit your face like your cheek bones, the bridge of your nose, chin, and forehead. Blush and bronze, like all the other details of your makeup, should look natural and like a part of your skin tone. Always apply lightly at first, check your face in natural light and then apply more, if needed.

SHAVING

The easiest way to shave your legs is in the bath or shower. The hot water and humidity opens the pores on your legs and enables you to get an extra-close shave, plus it will make your skin softer and more elastic to prevent nicks and cuts. Apply a good moisturizer after shaving, while your skin is still damp.

To avoid bumps and in-grown hairs, thoroughly cleanse and exfoliate the skin before shaving.

Remember, never share your razor, as it can spread infection. Always moisturize your skin immediately after shaving. Shave your legs daily for ultra-smooth skin. If you're using disposable razors, change them after about six shaves.

If you have run out of shaving cream, hair conditioner or baby/body oil can be a good substitute. Oil can also be used if you have no water available. If you find that the hair on your legs is becoming coarser, shave less often. There are hair inhibitors on the market that will soften and lighten your leg hair after a few weeks of use.

For facial hair, I recommend hot wax treatments. You can also use depilatory creams or gels specially formulated for the sensitive skin on your face. Be sure to always do a patch test first to ensure the treatment works well with your skin. If it causes irritation or any problems then use something else.

DEODORANTS

We all sweat and there's nothing wrong with that. But using the right items here can reduce the impact of it, like odors and damage to clothing.

Remember the difference: "antiperspirants" block sweat, while "deodorants" block odor by using fragrances.

Use a deodorant with antiperspirant for your best protection against odor and wetness. There are many types of deodorants and antiperspirants on the market today but those with aluminum chloride are the most effective at blocking sweat glands. For particularly troublesome sweat problems, apply your deodorant before bed, so it can absorb fully by the morning.

Experiment with different antiperspirants and deodorants to find the ones with the most active ingredients. Crystal deodorants are an interesting choice. To use them, you wet the crystal and then rub it on your armpits, releasing mineral salts that stop odor-causing bacteria.

Another tip is to wear light-colored clothes in natural fibers during the warmer months; these will help absorb sweat and avoid stains.

If you have sensitive skin, there are moisturizing deodorants on the market today that will be more soothing, and don't keep using a product if it causes you great irritation. There are also stronger, heavier-duty deodorants if you have a busy day ahead and need more protection.

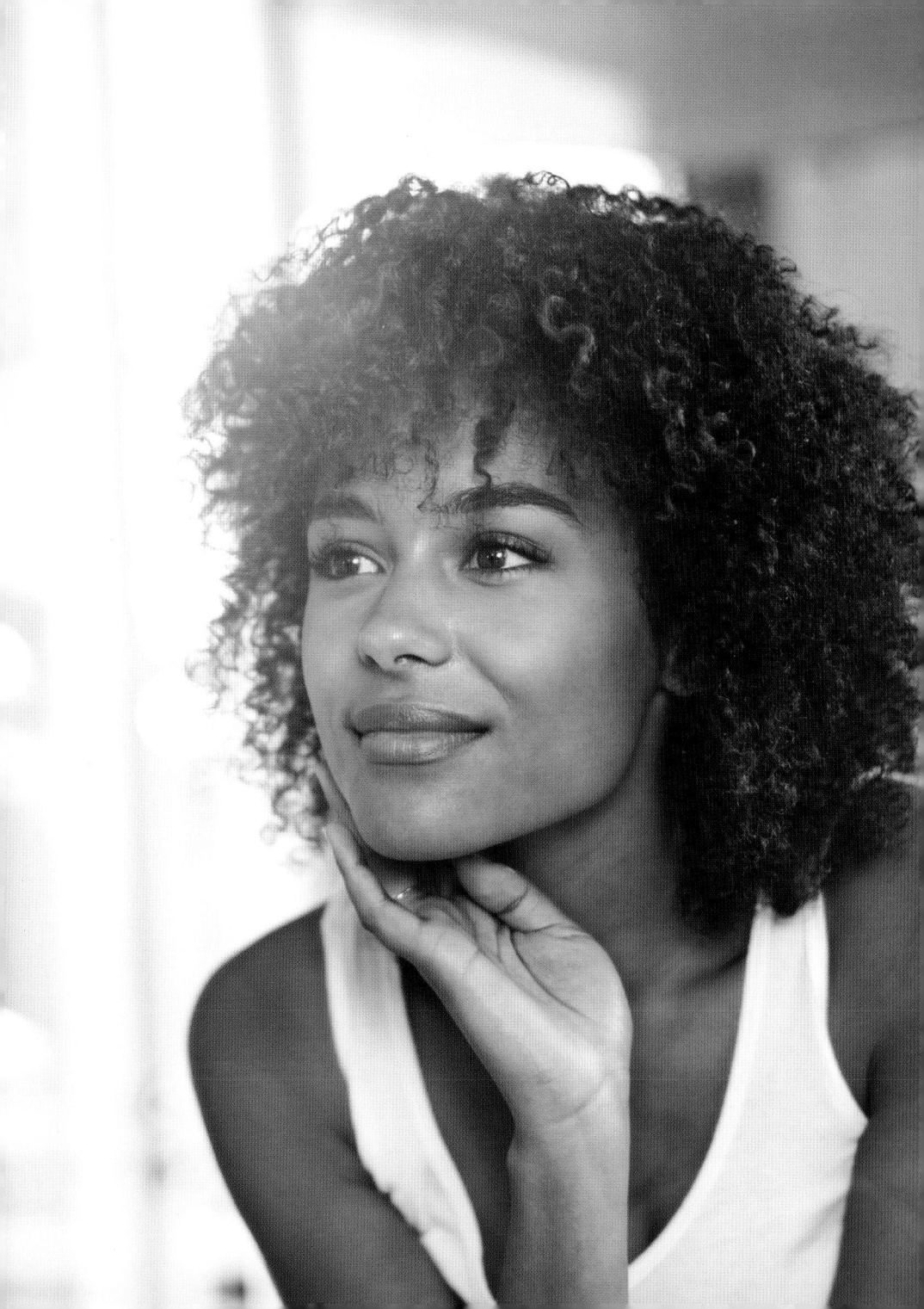

NAILS

Shorter nails are more stylish and easier to maintain. When I say short, I don't mean something you bit down to the nub—please don't even consider biting your nails. And if you are one of those women that bite your toe nails, please return this book to my home address for a full refund!

There's nothing wrong with giving yourself a manicure (it can save time and money). You just have to remember a few things:

III When giving yourself a manicure, always use a basecoat.

III Nail polish colors, especially the dark, vampy colors will stain your nails.

III Use two coats of polish. One coat will peel off too quickly and more than two coats will be too thick.

III Apply thin coats of polish and always finish with a top coat.

III A light shade of polish that blends in with your natural skin tone will give the appearance of longer, thinner hands.

III Short nails look better with very bright or very dark polish. Go with either a light and natural polish or a very dark color.

Allow thirty minutes for your nail polish to dry to avoid smudges, especially dark colors.

You might want to try a nail mask before your manicure to help moisturize your dry nails and cuticles. For a nail mask at home: warm up some oil, apply it to clean nails by gently massaging, and leave it on for at least an hour. Be sure to clean the oil off your nails completely before applying polish. Try essential oils, lavender, lemon, tea tree, olive, almond, or rosemary.

Every few weeks, leave your nails bare so they can breathe. Otherwise, have fun and experiment with your nails!

PEDICURE

Our feet all too often get forgotten. Here is a quick way to do a homemade pedicure.

Before bed each night apply a foot cream. Use one with large concentrations of exfoliate like salicylic acid and alpha hydroxyl acids. These exfoliants will soften the feet and make any rough skin baby soft.

Going barefoot occasionally around the house is good for your feet as it exercises the foot muscles.

When applying nail polish to your toenails, follow the same rules as I set out above.

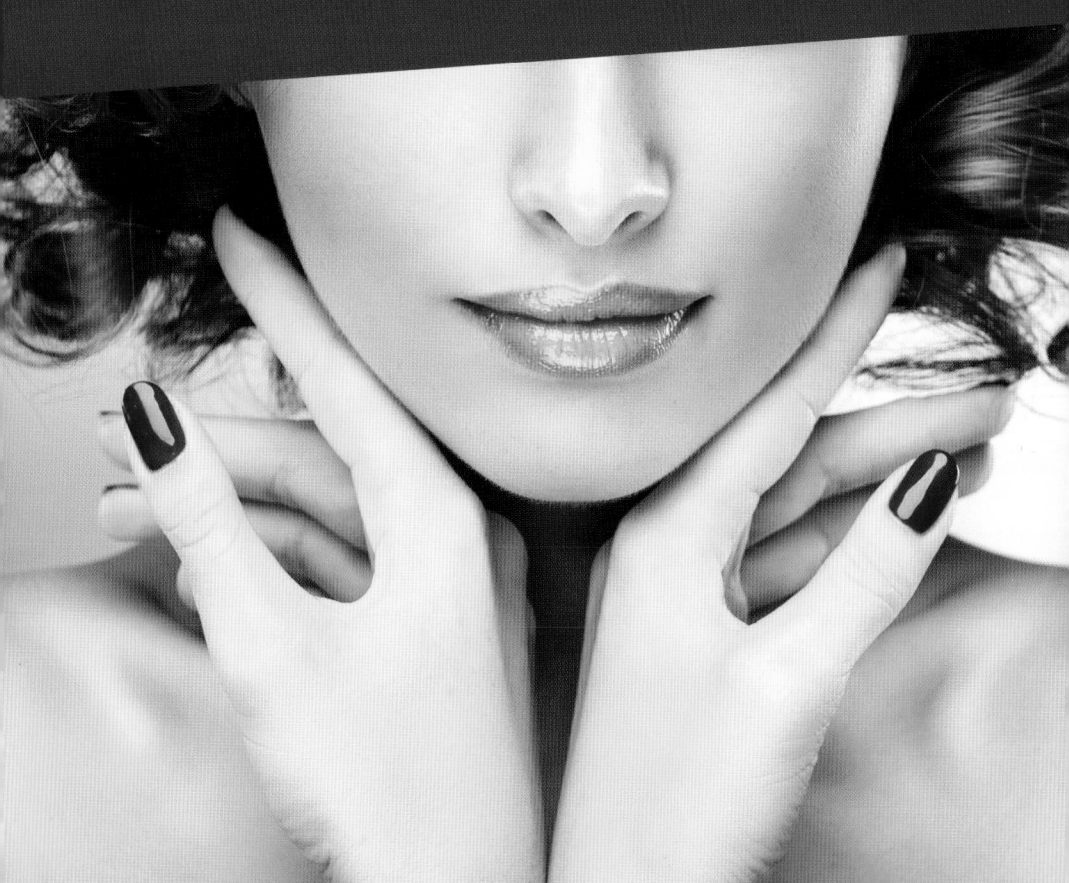

LONG, SHORT

& EVERYTHING IN BETWEEN

HOW TO TRULY CARE FOR YOUR HAIR

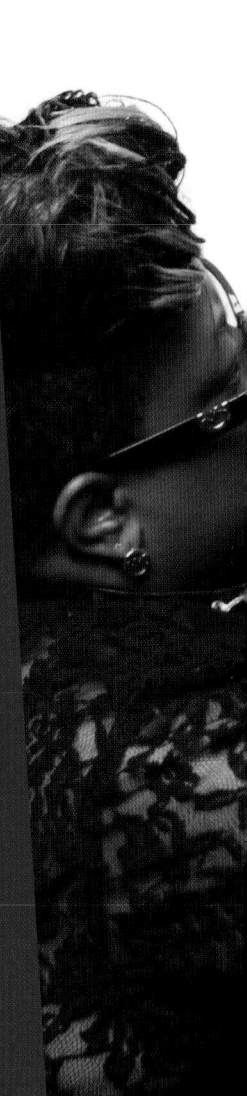

To say my hair has been "my thing" throughout my adult life and career is an understatement. From curly and dark, to blonde highlights and constant blow outs with flat iron finishing, I had to learn a thing or two about how to keep it healthy, shiny, and bouncy. Something that hasn't always been easy since there were weeks when I would sit to have it done three, four, and five times!

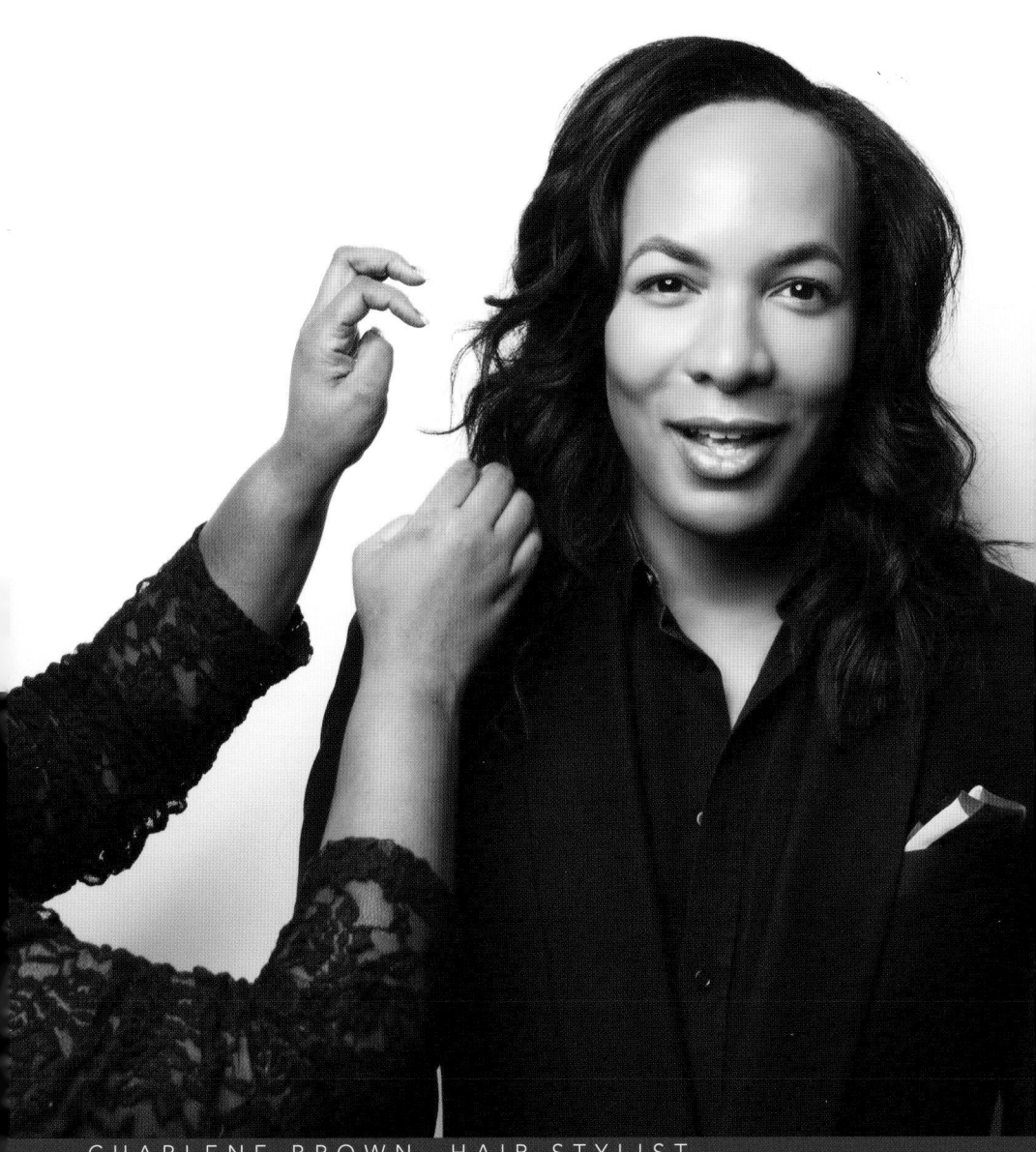

CHARLENE BROWN, HAIR STYLIST

Most people of a certain age have some kind of color worked into their hair, whether it be to cover grey hair, to highlight or to low light their natural color. If you want to experiment with color the key is to keep it looking fresh. To keep your new color treatment from fading, wash your hair with cool water, never hot. I know that sounds awful, but the cool water helps to seal in the cuticle and keep your hair from looking frizzy and rough.

Maintaining healthy hair has a lot to do with managing extreme conditions. Blow-dry your hair on a warm or even cool setting. Hair is very vulnerable when it's wet and is most prone to damage by heat and rough treatment. Wash your hair less often to retain moisture and to keep your color from fading. Use color protecting, moisturizing- or keratin-enriched shampoos and conditioners.

Whether or not you are using color, go easy on the hair products and the heat! Less is more. Overuse of styling products will just weigh your hair down. Remember, limp, greasy, heavy, and difficult hair is usually the result of too much product. Less is always better. So lightly apply gels, mousses, and sprays while gently working through your hair.

Residue buildup on your hair will leave it looking dry, limp, and lifeless. To reduce this buildup, use a clarifying shampoo on your hair once a week.

For extra lift and volume, hold your head upside down while you blow-dry it, concentrating on the roots. This will also increase blood flow to your head, stimulating your hair follicles. Move the dryer around your scalp and apply a light spray of hair spray.

To keep your look fresh and new, update your hairdo periodically. Experiment with different cuts, colors and styles. If you get your hair styled with heat once a week, you'll want to get a trim every 8-12 weeks.

A WORD ON PRODUCTS

While I tell you to use products lightly, just as important is finding the right ones for your hair. Some people swear by switching their shampoos and conditioners as the seasons change. My line of Paul Wharton Hair Care Products are enriched with Keratin and help the hair go from curly to straight with ease – products like these should work for you forever. It's important to buy products that are made for your type of hair; find what works for you.

I would advise you to only use two-in-one shampoos and conditioners for a short time. They don't have the specialized ingredients that you find in separate products that your hair needs on a regular basis.

Food makes a huge difference, believe it or not—a well-balanced diet will guarantee that the blood supplied to your hair follicles is full of nutrients. The overall condition of your hair will be determined by your general health and lifestyle and factors like: drinking, smoking, medication, age, and health. If you lead a healthy lifestyle, exercise, and eat healthy nutritious foods, your hair should reflect your good health and be healthy and glorious (see Chapter 4 in this book for some general advice).

If possible, don't start blow-drying until your hair is semi-dry. On wet hair, first apply mousse or gel to hold your style, then a gel or serum to keep it smooth. For shine plus hold, spray your hairbrush with hairspray and brush through your hair, all the way to the ends.

Always hold a blow dryer at least six inches from your scalp and vary the temperature settings, using high heats only for short intervals. If your hair is oily or greasy, always blow-dry your hair on a cool setting. Hot air will cause your oil glands to increase production of sebum.

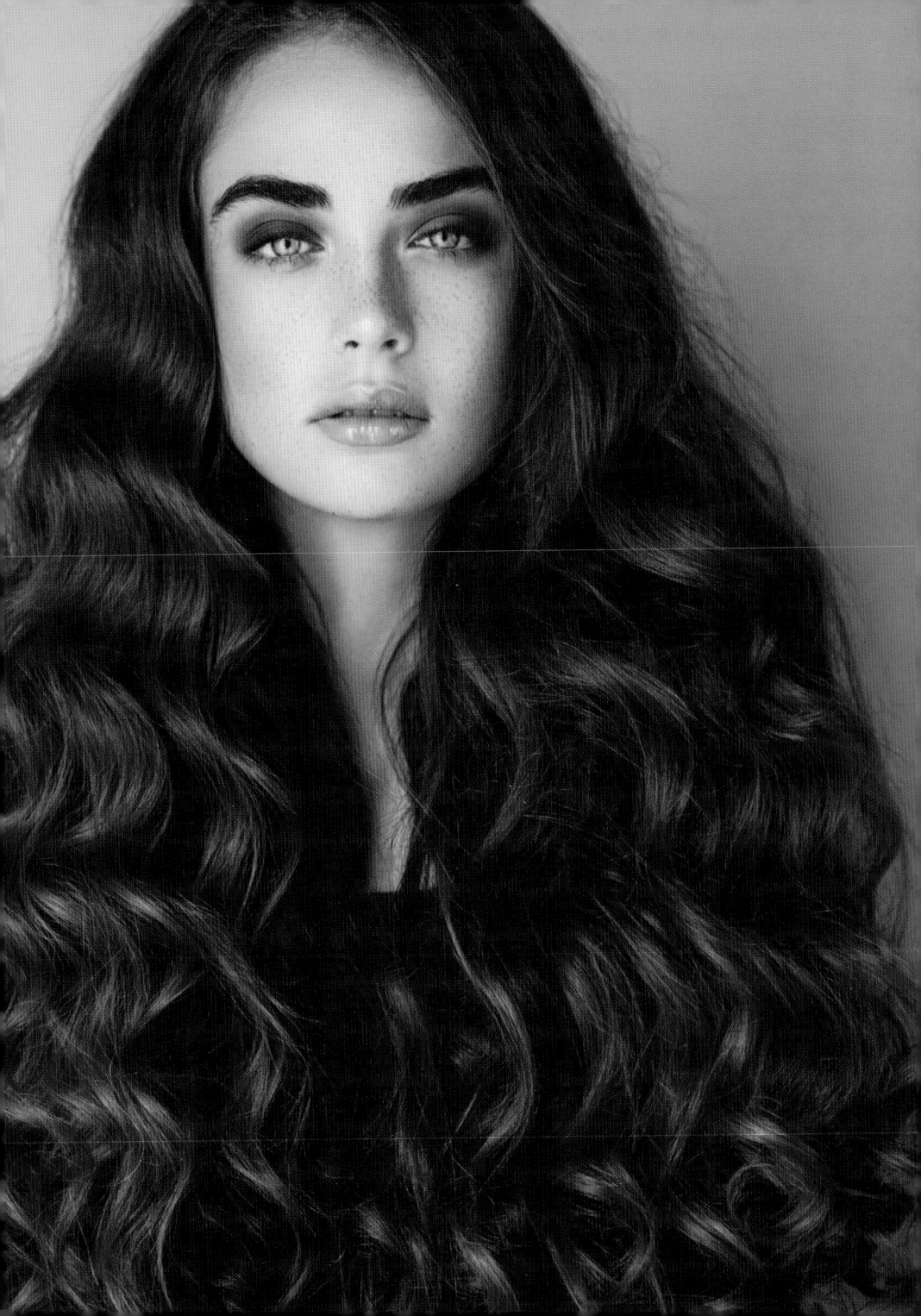

If your hair is badly damaged, try conditioning your hair before you shampoo, in addition to your regular routine. You may need to use more than one type of conditioner. Use a color-enhancing conditioner if you have color. It will keep your hair looking fresh and prevent the color from fading too quickly. Alternate your conditioners in order to address all of your hair issues.

Use leave-in conditioner for African-American hair to give curls shine and separation. It is healthier and dries the hair out less when you use leave-in conditioner on your hair in place of styling gels and sprays.

Paul's Expert Tip

Although there are hundreds of hair care products on the market today, none can repair split ends, so stop holding on to them. Get your stylist to trim the ends and have your hair trimmed regularly to keep them from reappearing.

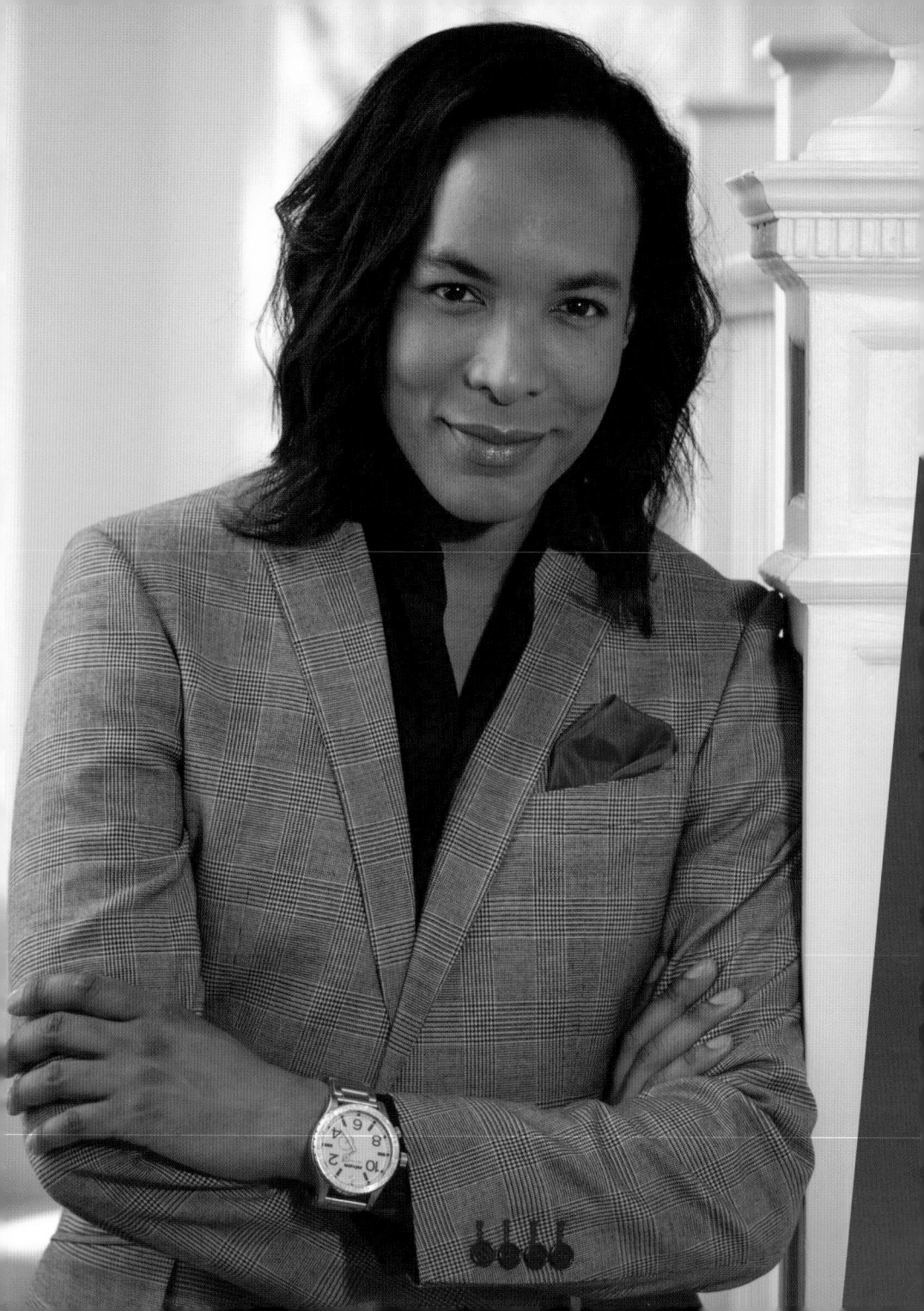

PAUL'S LAST WORD

I'm going to repeat my opening in this chapter—makeup and haircare can be great, it can be fun, and make you feel more confident. But I don't want you to think that you need to spend hours on your face or that there's anything wrong with skipping makeup altogether if you don't have time or don't feel like it.

Believe me when I tell you that you're perfect and beautiful—makeup and haircare are all ways to enhance what you already have, so don't think of it as trying to change the way you look altogether.

I WANT YOU TO
LOVE
YOURSELF
AND USE MY ADVICE
IN THE RIGHT WAY

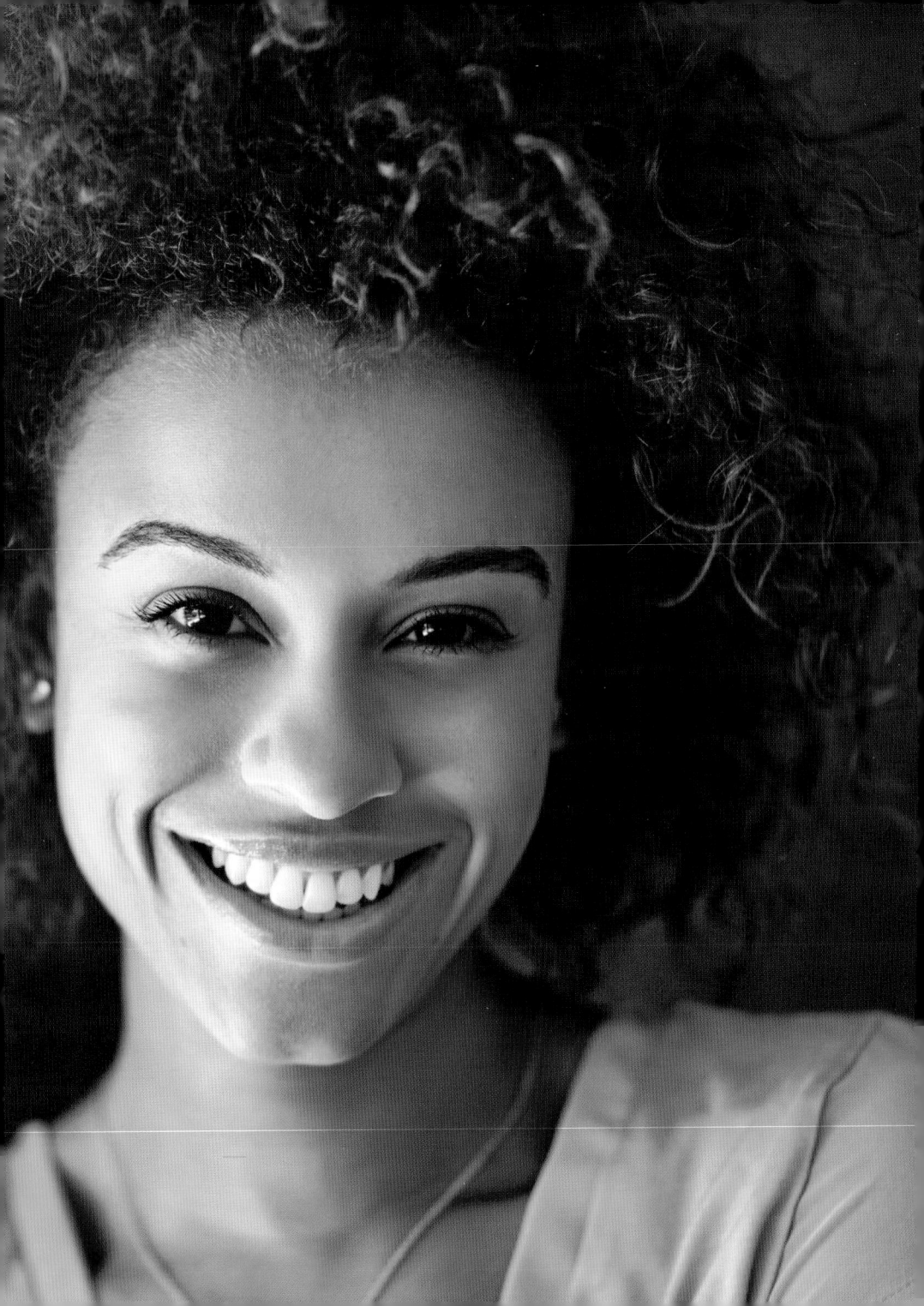

CHAPTER 3

SKIN
DEEP

AN EFFICIENT & EFFECTIVE
SKINCARE ROUTINE

When I was younger I suffered from very bad acne—it impacted my career, my personal life, and above all else, my confidence. I spent a fortune on every treatment I could find over the years and saw doctor after doctor.

Eventually, I began to research everything myself. I looked into the products and treatments I was using, learning the science and trying to understand what was good and bad. After a while I realized that some of products out there on the market aren't that great for your skin—many of them have ingredients which can dry out or even irritate your skin, or which are only suitable for specific skin types. After a lot of work I managed to find treatments that really worked for me and I am lucky to have clear skin again.

Inspired by my experience and because I really want to help other people who have had the same problems, I developed my own line of skincare products, the Paul Wharton Beauty range. The key for me was to create something which could be effective for most skin types and was simple enough that busy people can fit it into their lives without having to compromise.

So here is my five-step skincare routine—you probably do one, two, or maybe even three of the steps, but I wanted to share my experience of the products themselves and advise some extra things that you may want to try to enhance your routine.

CLEANSE

Your daily skin-care regimen should start with finding a cleanser that is right for you. You need to look for a product that exfoliates the skin and removes excess oils and impurities for a smoother, clearer complexion.

I use natural derivatives of active ingredients in my Paul Wharton Beauty line of products. My pore detox cleanser uses white willow bark, a natural source of salicylic acid to deeply penetrate each pore and gently exfoliate congested cells that build up and lead to blemishes and breakouts. Witch hazel, calendula extract, and tea tree oil also assist in purifying and soothing skin to encourage healing, reduce redness, and minimize the appearance of enlarged pores. In your product search, be sure to search look for added humectants, and the exclusion of sulfates. It is important to take out all of the bacteria and pore-blocking oils and debris without over drying or stripping your skin of its essential pH balance.

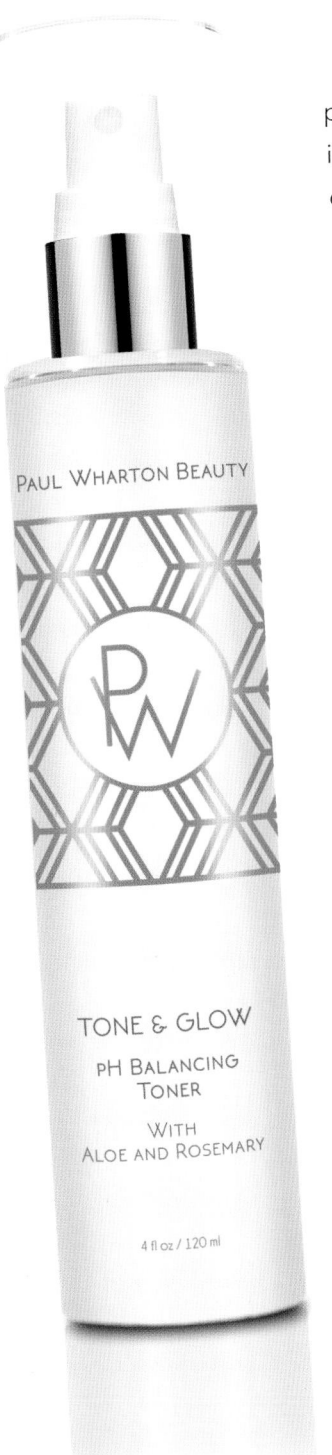

PAUL WHARTON BEAUTY

TONE & GLOW

pH BALANCING
TONER

WITH
ALOE AND ROSEMARY

4 fl oz / 120 ml

When I was in my teens and early twenties, I used products that were designed to combat acne. If acne is also a problem for you, then look for gentle foaming cleansers as these should work well without being too harsh on your skin.

TONE

I guarantee that you've seen toners in-store, you may even own and use them. But I still think a majority of people are unclear on exactly what a toner does and why you should use it—well, your friend Paul is here to help out.

In a sentence, a toner is a product which helps to replenish and hydrate your skin after cleansing and it can also help to remove the last remnants of dust, makeup, and other elements which could remain after cleansing.

To give you a little more detail, a good toner (and I emphasize the word "good") will immediately hydrate your skin after cleansing and deliver vitamins and nourishment. The effect is to make your skin look instantly better and to significantly help repair and protect the skin. It can be used even without cleansing to give your skin a boost of hydration as well.

My Paul Wharton Beauty Tone and Glow toner is great for most skin types and loaded with potent botanical extracts like sea kelp, cucumber, sage, rosemary, orange, chamomile, allantoin, and aloe, plus Vitamin C and water-binding humectants like hyaluronic acid and Vitamin B5. It is specifically designed to soothe, heal, and rejuvenate your skin while providing anti-inflammatory, antioxidant, and bacterial benefits.

Applying toners is simple—after you cleanse, apply toner either to cotton pads or to your hands, and press onto the skin on your face and neck (always remember not to apply directly to your eyes). You can even apply during the day when your skin feels like it needs a boost of moisture and hydration.

There are different kinds of toner and always remember to consider your own skin type. But unless you have very oily skin or a particular medical need, I would recommend staying clear of very astringent toners—these are ones which often have a lot of alcohol and other ingredients that are harsh for skin.

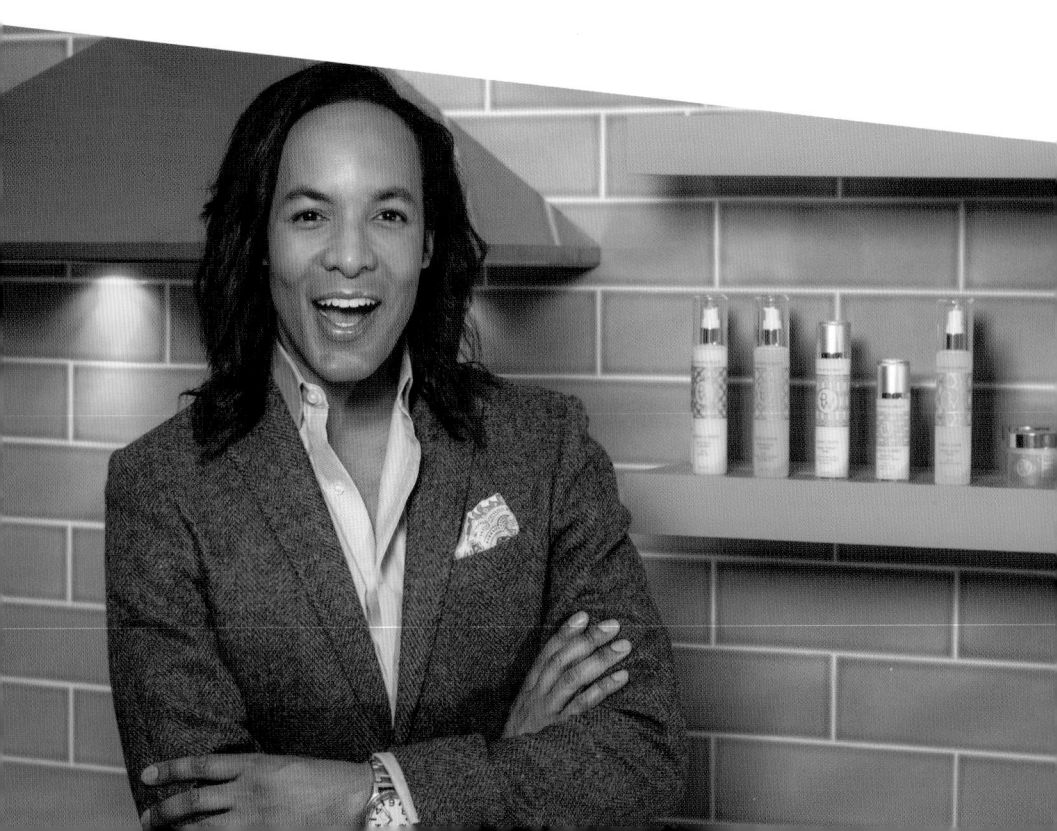

MOISTURIZE

I'm sure I don't need to explain to you about why a moisturizer is so important. I have yet to meet a lady who has never used one and I rarely meet someone who doesn't have at least three or four different moisturizers in their bathroom.

So I'm not going to lecture you on the importance of this step, but I will tell you what you should be getting out of your product. There are so many different types of moisturizer and they all promise to fix everything and turn back time—the truth is that the right ones can actually reverse some of aging process. But there are lot of fakers on the market.

It's easy to get really drawn into the science here, but let's keep it big-picture. Firstly, we all know that hydration is important and that your moisturizer should contain ingredients which are going to add moisture (hence the product name). So you want to avoid products with lots of alcohol and chemicals which may dry out the skin over time and you want to find a product that will help to seal after application so that it also keeps the moisture from dissipating.

Paul's Expert Tip

If you find that a regular moisturizer is too heavy for your skin, consider trying a good toner in place of your moisturizer in the morning. It won't give you everything the moisturizer can, but it will hydrate and protect your skin without making it more oily. I would still advise that you use a moisturizer at night before sleep to really replenish everything, but in the day, this might help you stay hydrated while keeping your complexion clear.

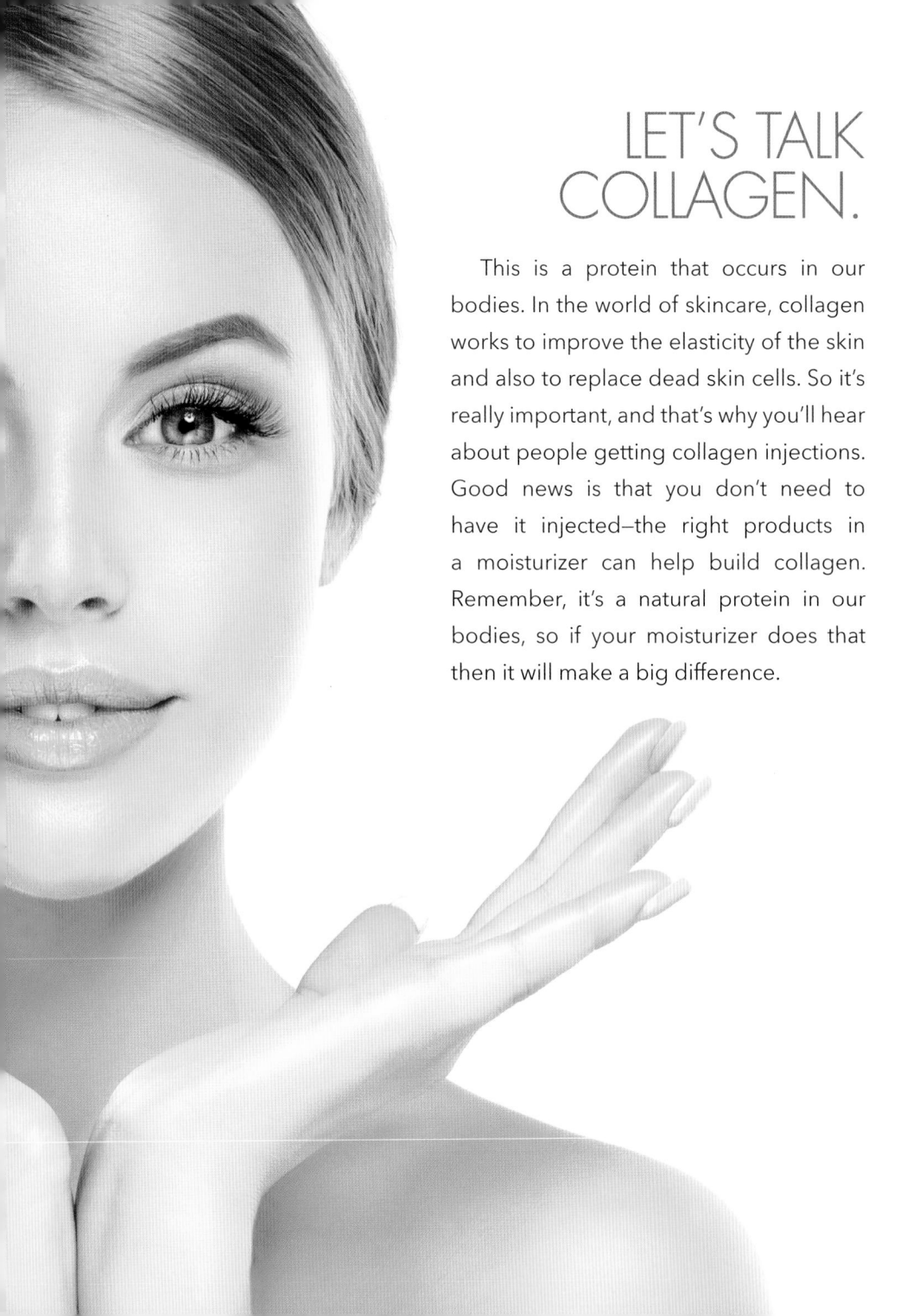

LET'S TALK COLLAGEN.

This is a protein that occurs in our bodies. In the world of skincare, collagen works to improve the elasticity of the skin and also to replace dead skin cells. So it's really important, and that's why you'll hear about people getting collagen injections. Good news is that you don't need to have it injected—the right products in a moisturizer can help build collagen. Remember, it's a natural protein in our bodies, so if your moisturizer does that then it will make a big difference.

My Paul Wharton Beauty Botanic Youth Global Therapy Crème includes Vitamin C, ferulic acid, and algae extracts with specialized amino acids, phospholipids, and botanicals to hydrate, protect, and support melanin and collagen production. All the things you need for your skin, but I kept it light so won't make you greasy.

EXFOLIATE

I'm going to keep this section really simple for y'all—exfoliation is very important but it's equally important not to overdo it. We all know that dead skin cells need to be scrubbed or brushed away and this causes the skin to speed up cell production. We all know that doing this will keep our complexion more even and balanced, and we all know that exfoliating is the way to do it.

You can use exfoliating products several times a week but be careful not to overdo it. A mistake I find women make is exfoliating everyday with a harsh scrub, which can dry out your skin. Technically, once a week is enough, but a few times a week is good so long as you are using the right product.

So the easy part is this: find a good exfoliator and use it at least once a week as part of your regimen. The great news is that the exfoliating product will last for a long time.

The hard part (as with so much of skincare) is finding the right product. There are lots of harsh exfoliating products out there; clearing dead skin cells does not mean you have scrub your face raw or dry it out. The right product can help to clean and also nourish without feeling rough.

For the Paul Wharton Beauty range I created the Revive and Reveal Exfoliating Micro Derm Scrub which includes micro-crystals to gently sweep away the dead cells and debris but also filled it with antioxidants to help revive your skin at the same time.

If you choose manual exfoliants, choose one with small beads or grains that you can massage gently. If you choose a chemical exfoliant, a glycolic or alpha hydroxyl acid, apply for the recommended time (never longer) and rinse off.

Combination skin can use most exfoliants, since it is sometimes dry and sometimes oily. However, you always want to use a gentle scrub or an exfoliant with enzymes and small fine grains.

Word of advice—if your T-zone is oily, consider using a special mask for that area. If your skin is very dry and dehydrated, use a moisturizer that has hyaluronic acid.

CHOOSE AN EXFOLIANT FOR YOUR SKIN TYPE:

▐▐ Dry and sensitive skin types need gentle exfoliation so the calming and soothing creams you apply will go to work. Use a cream exfoliant that contains natural fruit enzymes to gently remove the dead cells. Get soothing masks with aloe, hyaluronic, and calming extracts.

▐▐ Oily skin needs exfoliation to remove the dead skin cells that are clogging up the pores and causing breakouts. Choose a scrub with soft scrubbing beads and fine grains. Use an exfoliant with a mild salicylic acid solution to help unclog pores. After exfoliating, use a moisturizer, especially for oily skin, that contains calming ingredients to prevent redness.

▐▐ If you are using concentrated acne products or anti-aging products always apply to dry skin. Let the product absorb for ten minutes, then apply moisturizer.

The best way to incorporate exfoliation is to keep it simple and replace the cleansing part of your routine with an exfoliating scrub. If the product is good then you only need a dime-sized amount. Apply it to a clean damp face and neck and massage gently in circular motions. You should not need to scrub hard. And as always, avoid the skin around the eye area—the tissue around the eyes is very sensitive.

When you exfoliate then always do it before moisturizing, not after. The dead skin cells need to be sloughed off before the moisturizer can be absorbed. Rinse thoroughly after application and then follow the rest of your regimen with toner and apply moisturizer to damp skin for the most effective absorption.

REPAIR

We spend a lot of time and money on our faces—let's be honest, this is mainly because we want to look good. But it's also the part of our body that takes the most damage because it's the most exposed. The rest of our bodies get covered up regularly. But the face is always out there, even when we're sleeping with the covers pulled up, our face is sitting out there. When you think about how much our faces take every day from the sun, wind, rain, changes in temperature, drying out from air conditioning, to sweating when we work out, it's only logical that we put some effort into protecting it.

This brings me to my final step in the skincare regime: how to repair our skin after all it's done for us. This is a step which a lot of people tend to skip, as it's often seen as an add-on or an extra product. So I have put it last, because if you cleanse, tone, moisturize, and repair as I advised before, your skin is going to be in good shape.

But this is actually a very simple extra step—it takes only a few seconds extra and is easy to work into your routine: using a repair serum.

Quick note: a serum has smaller molecules than a moisturizer and so it can penetrate deeper and really push those healing ingredients and hydration deep into your skin.

Remember I talked about "free radicals" in the Cleanse section, and the importance of collagen in the Moisturize section? Well, a good serum will both neutralize the free radicals and help prevent the breakdown of collagen. When looking at repair serums, try to find one that will target these things, like my Paul Wharton Beauty Defend & Correct Serum which has age-defying antioxidants to really protect and repair your skin.

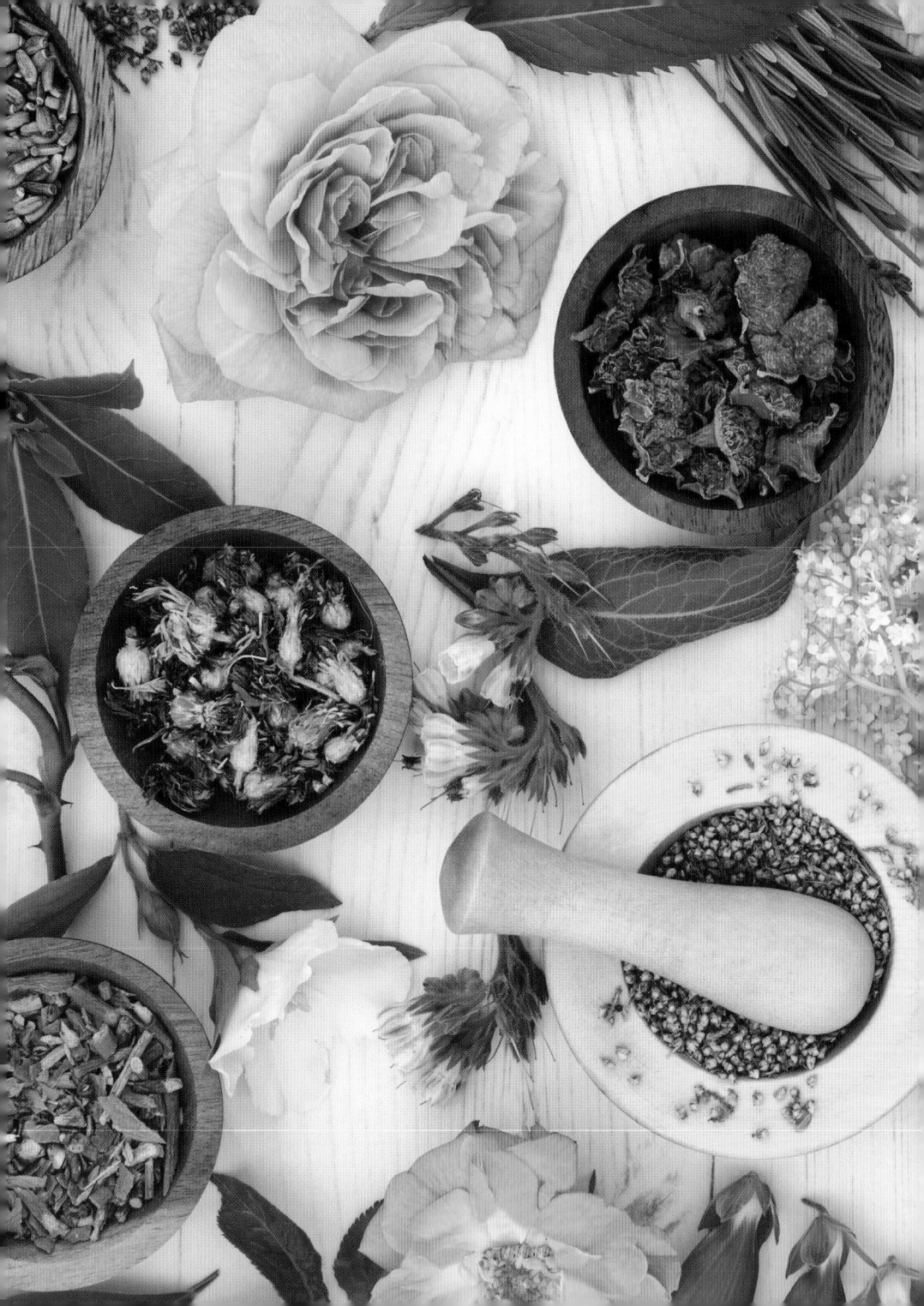

When you choose a serum, it is worth spending a little more because you should use it sparingly. After cleansing and toning, add a drop (that really is all you need) to your forehead, chin, and cheeks, and massage in gently. Then apply moisturizer.

While it is not essential,

I STRONGLY RECOMMEND ADDING A REPAIR SERUM TO YOUR ROUTINE.

It can boost your regimen and once again it won't take a lot of extra time.

Paul's Expert Tip

You can make your own exfoliator. I love to use a little white granulate to exfoliate my skin. Start with two teaspoons of sugar, add a gentle facial cleanser and warm water. Mix it in the palms of your hands, and gently massage onto your face in a circular motion. Rinse with warm water and finish with a refreshing toner.

A WORD
ON ANTI-AGING

I started incorporating anti-aging skin care into my personal regimen when I was in my mid- to late twenties by moving completely away from the harsh, clear-the-bumps-by-any-means-necessary products that most of the time left my skin feeling dry and looking gray and dull. It's never too early to start and cleansing is a critical part. If you're over the age of twenty-five, you should start an anti-aging regimen and continue to follow it over the next fifty years!

Here's a little science for you—"free radicals," as they are referred to, are your enemy in the fight against premature aging. Free radicals can be found in alcohol, fried foods, pesticides, air pollutants, and excessive exposure to the sun. They can cause damage to parts of cells such as proteins, DNA, and cell membranes by stealing their electrons through a process called oxidation. So, to keep our skin looking fresh, we must reverse the damaging effects of free radicals and replenish all that has been diminished through our skin's exposure to the enemy.

My Paul Wharton Beauty line's anti-aging cleanser is a sulfate-free, foaming daily anti-aging cleanser that delivers powerful antioxidants to the skin to protect and repair, while gentle alpha hydroxy acids hydrate, exfoliate, and smooth away uneven texture caused by intrinsic aging. Catechin-rich green tea & white tea extracts help fortify skin's cellular matrix, defending against free radical damage and helping to prevent collagen breakdown. Many of us have seen the hollow look become an issue and this is due to the skin's loss of collagen. It is easier to preserve the collagen than to rebuild it, so that's why it's so important to get started early. Lactic acid also works synergistically with these antioxidants and other humectants to increase dermal glycosaminoglycan (support of collagen) content and normalize hyperkeratinization (dead skin cells trapped in a follicle), exfoliating away dead skin cells that contribute to uneven skin texture and a dull complexion.

The point of finding the proper cleansers and exfoliants for your skin is to repair and prep skin for the delivery and optimal penetration of companion anti-aging products. The products that do the real repair work, the heavy lifting! Without a good cleanser, your moisturizer and other products are not going to be nearly as effective.

A final word on acne: even if you don't face the type of acne that I did, we all break out sometimes. A quick and easy way to eliminate blackheads is using pore strips. Apply the pore strips to the affected area, smooth it out, and wait for fifteen minutes before removing the strip. You can buy them specially formulated for your nose, forehead, and chin.

Paul's Expert Tip

If your knees and elbows are discolored and rough, try mixing the juice from a lemon, a bit of sugar for spreading consistency, and apply the mixture to areas where needed. Leave on for two to three minutes. Rub off with a warm wash cloth, and apply moisturizer for smoother skin. Do this on a regular basis to get through the tough outer layer of skin.

A WORD ON MASKS

The reason that masks don't get their own section in this book is that I want you to keep a skincare regime that is simple and achievable. If you make things too complex, you are more likely to let it slide and stop following it. But masks can be a useful addition so I have included a few words here because I think they work at their best after exfoliation or cleansing.

Before applying a mask, cleanse your face, then rinse well with lukewarm water. Apply the mask generously, according to the label instructions

AS ALWAYS, CHOOSE A MASK SUITABLE FOR YOUR SKIN TYPE:

- III For dry skin, use a clay or mud mask; for oily skin, use a creamy one with aloe or lavender and chamomile to boost the moisture content.

- III For sensitive skin, be very careful choosing a mask. Use a very gentle mask with calming, soothing ingredients.

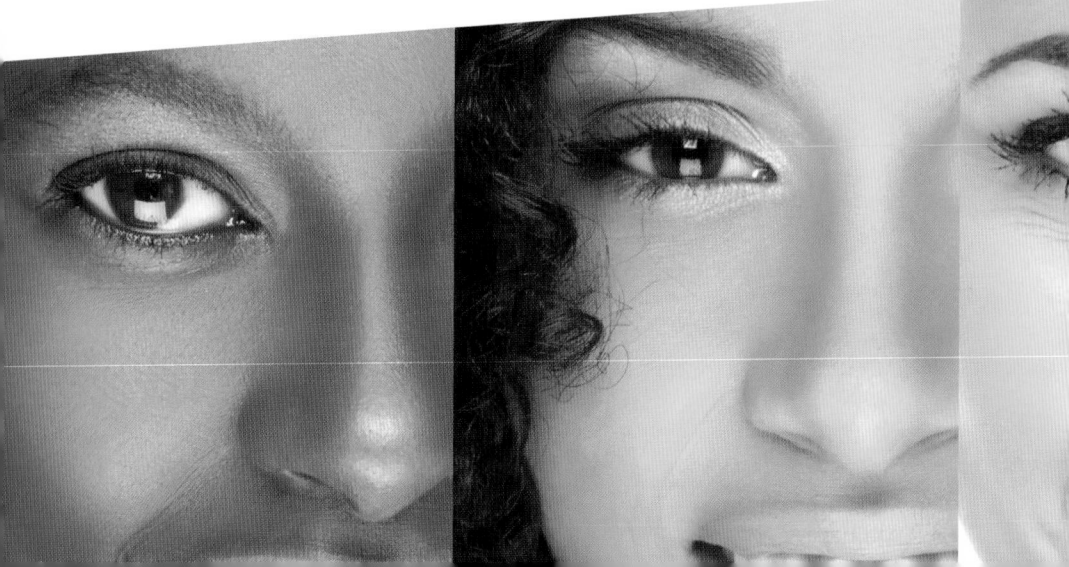

Rinse off the mask, tone, and apply a moisturizer for your skin type while your skin is still damp.

Lie down and put your feet up while you're waiting for your mask to work its magic. Relax and enjoy all the benefits of a little pampering. This will increase the circulation of blood and oxygen from the lower body to your face and the mask will be more absorbent and effective.

Masks are not just for your face, they can be used on your body and wherever your skin needs a little extra help: your legs, shoulders, or feet. Generously apply the type of mask needed (clay, seaweed, etc.) for your problem area. Allow the mask to dry, and then hop in the shower, rinse off, and moisturize. Dermatologists recommend using a mask that contains ingredients that have natural antibiotic properties like sulfur to help prevent further flare-ups.

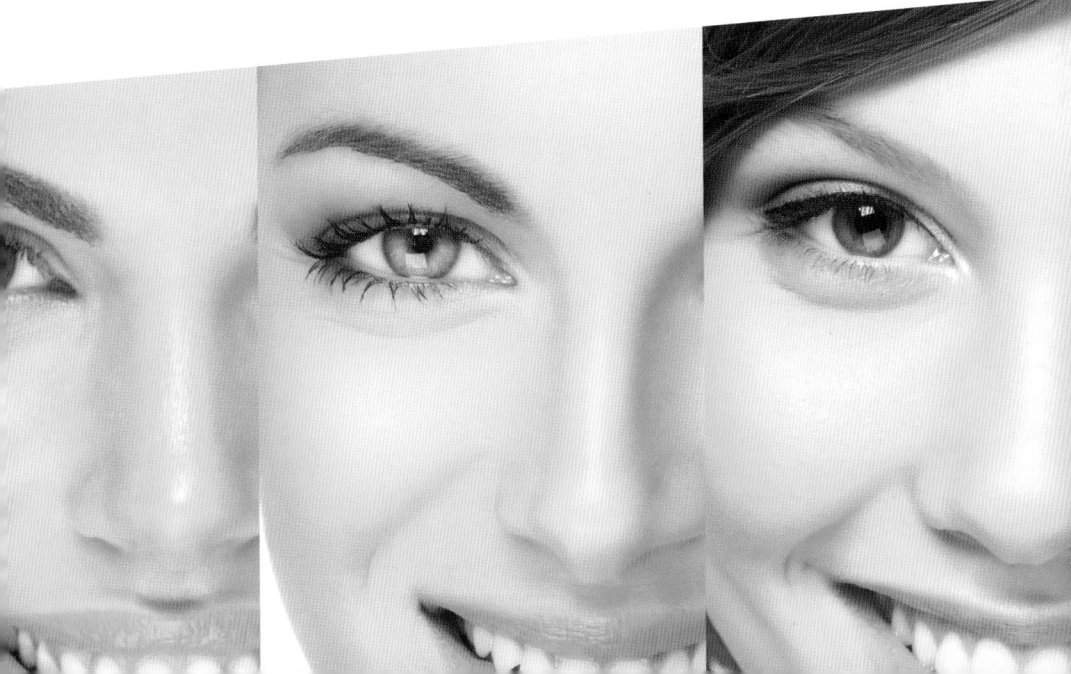

BODY

Many people treat their faces on a daily basis but when it comes to their bodies, not so much. Beauty extends beyond your chin and it's important not to neglect the rest of our bodies. Here a few pieces of advice that I have found make a big difference:

III Don't forget to apply sunscreen on the top of your feet and all the way to the toes before hitting the beach or pool (or just when you're wearing sandals outside). The tops of your feet take a direct hit from the sun and will show signs of aging, just like the rest of your body.

III Knees are a sure sign of age. Keep them looking youthful by dry brushing, exfoliating, and using emollient-rich moisturizers regularly.

III Your chest and neck should be included in your daily skin care regime. Use the gentle cleanser you use on your face and moisturizer that contains antioxidants when you exfoliate your face, continue to the neck and chest area to remove dead skin cells and any damaged skin.

III Find a hand cream that has a sunscreen in it and apply it every time you wash your hands. Your hands are exposed to every kind of element and abuse and need protection, especially from sun damage. Exfoliate your hands and arms and then use an antioxidant-enriched moisturizer. This will help seal in moisture and help prevent chipped and broken nails.

III Stretch marks occur when your skin can't deal with the rapid expansion of extra flesh under the skin. They are permanent, although over time they can fade and become less obvious. If you keep your skin well-moisturized, you may be able to fend off any new ones. After bathing, while your skin is still moist, apply a luxurious moisturizer and allow it to penetrate and absorb before dressing.

III Hands and feet are two places that are most forgotten. Use super moisturizing formulas that contain nourishing essential oils and some exfoliating agents. You can use high-tech rich, ultra-hydrating moisturizers on both your hands and feet.

- Read the ingredients on the sunscreens available today. These face and body protectors have intense moisturizers built into them and antioxidants to protect against free radicals while protecting your skin from harmful rays.

- If your skin tends to be oily, look for an oil-free sunscreen that won't clog your pores.

- Use the same scrubs, exfoliants, and enzymes on your body that you use on your face. Body scrubs with grains have moisturizing ingredients in them and are made specifically for your particular skin type.

- Don't forget the skin on your knees and elbows. This skin tends to be thicker and needs regular exfoliation and rich moisturizers. If that skin is especially dry and flaky, use a lotion that contains an alpha hydroxyl acid.

- Your neck and breast areas are especially sensitive areas, since they lack fat tissue. They can be the first to show visible signs of aging. Use the same rich anti-aging cleansers and moisturizers on your neck that you use on your face, instead of harsh soaps. Facial products have more concentrated nourishing ingredients in them and will work well on these areas. There are special creams and lotions available for these areas, too.

- Dry brushing your skin is a great way to get your circulation going, remove dead skin cells, fight cellulite, and make your skin smooth and glowing. It's best to dry brush before your morning shower. Use a soft washcloth or a long handle brush and start from your feet and work your way up towards your heart. Start with light brush strokes and as you progress into a daily routine, add more pressure. You will feel invigorated and notice moister, smoother skin in just a few days.

- Treat yourself to a professional full-body massage. There's nothing better for your mind and body. A body massage will release beneficial chemicals throughout your body and boost energy levels as well as activate your central nervous system, by stimulating your circulation. The increase in circulation can lower your blood pressure, making you feel relaxed and de-stressed. Get one as often as you can afford it.

DARKER SKIN

For darker brown skin tones, when your skin gets dry, it can look grayish or ashy, so you may need to take a few extra steps.

Washing too vigorously can remove too many of the natural oils in your skin, leaving your skin dry and tight. Use a gentle cleanser that's not too drying. Avoid cleansers with any abrasive granules in them; they can cause skin irritations, enlarged pores, and even broken capillaries. Treat your beautiful brown skin gently. After washing, pat dry, never rub or scrub or use harsh washcloths.

Dark skin needs special care and gentle handling to avoid any scarring, rashes, bruising, tearing, and hyper pigmentation. Many outside influences like overexposure to sunlight, scratches, and blemishes, can trigger your body to over or under produce melanin, causing discolorations of abnormal pigmentation. Black women should not try to treat their skin problems themselves: see a dermatologist. Most skin problems can be easily resolved if treated correctly by a professional. Otherwise, self-medicating can cause permanent damage.

Dark skin needs to be exfoliated just like any other type of skin, especially those with oily skin. The dead skin cells that block pores need to be removed to make way for the fresh new skin. Because of the susceptibility of brown skin scarring, always use a gentle exfoliate; again, nothing with harsh granules.

Use a skin cleanser that's formulated for your skin type (oily, dry, etc.), one that's thorough enough to remove all your makeup yet gentle enough for your delicate skin.

Women with darker skin have more melanin, which protects the skin. But melanin also blocks some skin treatments from penetrating deep into the skin. As long as you wash and rinse thoroughly, most botanical-based products these days will work just fine with brown skin, especially the ones with natural ingredients.

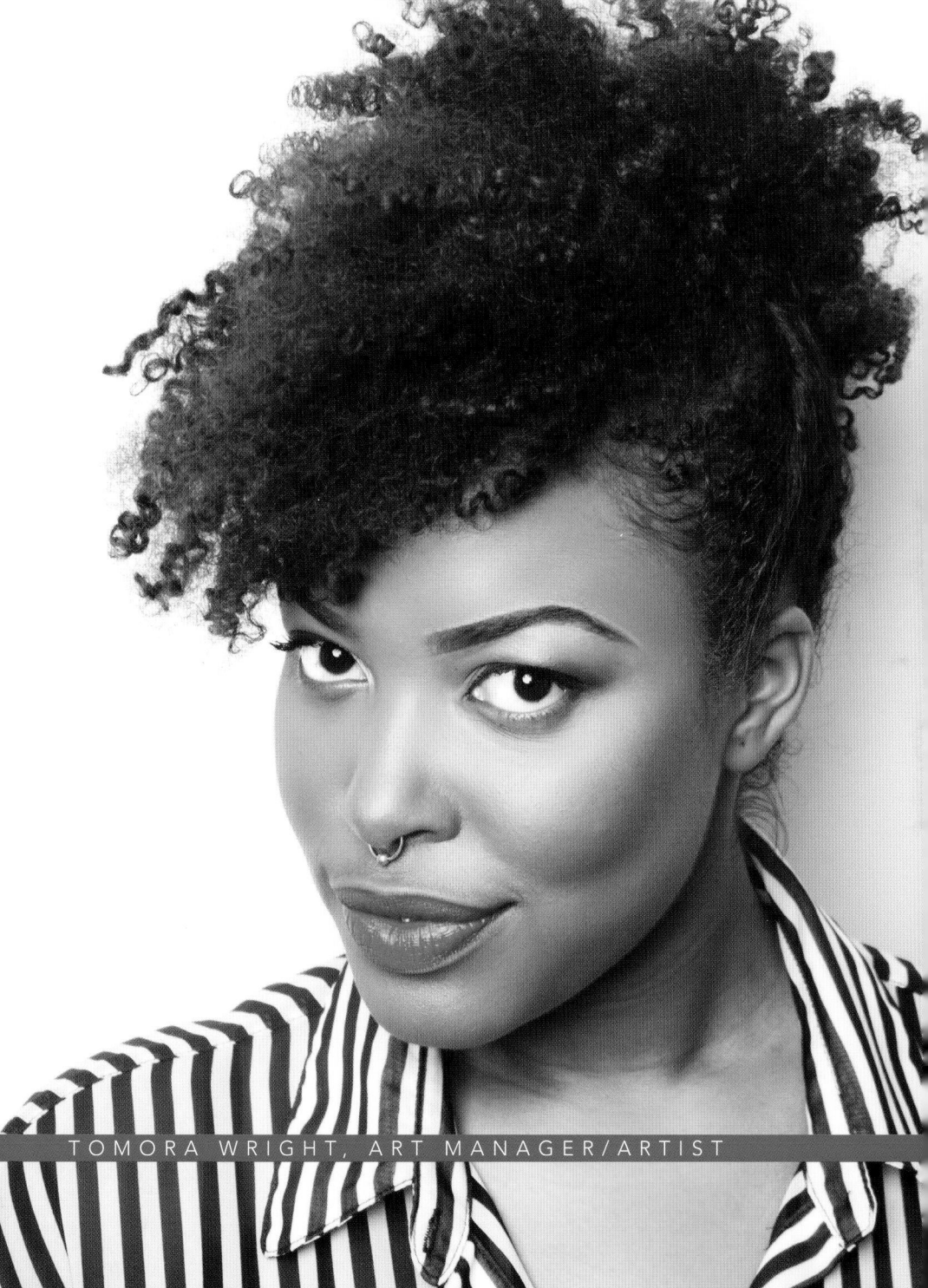
TOMORA WRIGHT, ART MANAGER/ARTIST

FEET

If you frequently wear high heels, you might want to visit a podiatrist. Most women wear the wrong size shoe. This can be very painful and cause bunions, hammertoes, and other painful foot ailments. A podiatrist can determine the correct size shoe you need, and help you with any other foot problems, and most insurance companies cover the visit.

Your feet get a lot of abuse in the summer, so give them a little extra TLC. Feet and legs have little or no oil glands and need to be moisturized. Exfoliate and moisturize them every day. Use a scrub in the shower—and then apply several layers of rich, creamy lotion. Put on some socks so the moisturizer will soak in, leaving your feet soft and smooth.

Carry a pack of handy wipes with you when wearing sandals or flip-flops, so you can keep your feet clean.

In the summer, when your feet are constantly on display, you'll need a pedicure every two or three weeks. Neutral and nude shades on your toes will allow you the most flexibility with your shoes and outfits.

If you're doing your own pedicure, buff out any discoloration, apply ridge filler, base coat, and a top coat.

Reapply a top coat every other day to prolong your pedicure, keep nails from chipping, and keep your toes looking shiny.

THE ART OF THE BATH

Pamper yourself after a long, exhausting day with a skin-smoothing, softening, and mood-enhancing bath. Set a relaxing mood by lighting some scented candles to create a warm glow. Put on some soothing music, unplug your phone, and put a do-not-disturb sign on the door. But here's how to do it right and make the most of your "me time" for your body and your skin.

A hot bath may sound relaxing, but a warm bath will be better for your skin and won't tire you out. You may want to stay in your bath all night but limit it to twenty minutes, at most. Add some bath and Epsom salts to soften the water and soothe tired and sore muscles. These minerals absorb into the skin and relieve your muscles as you soak.

For dry skin, add some apple cider vinegar or wine vinegar. Mix dry powered milk with water and add to your running bath water for a great moisturizer. Add a few drops of your favorite essential oil, depending on your mood. Essential oils do not always mix well so you'll want to mix a few drops in honey or cream before pouring into the tub for better absorption. Add the oils after you run your bathwater for maximum effectiveness.

Whenever possible, substitute a quick shower with a relaxing bath. But when a shower is all you have time for, buy some sinfully scented bath gels and sugared scrubs. Give yourself a mini-massage, or use a loofah and bath brush to increase your circulation. When you get out of the shower, dry off and apply some rich creamy lotions and moisturizers.

This is a great time to apply a facial mask. Use a clay mask to purify and cleanse oily skin, a hydrating, super-rich mask for dry skin, or an exfoliating mask to brighten and tighten the skin.

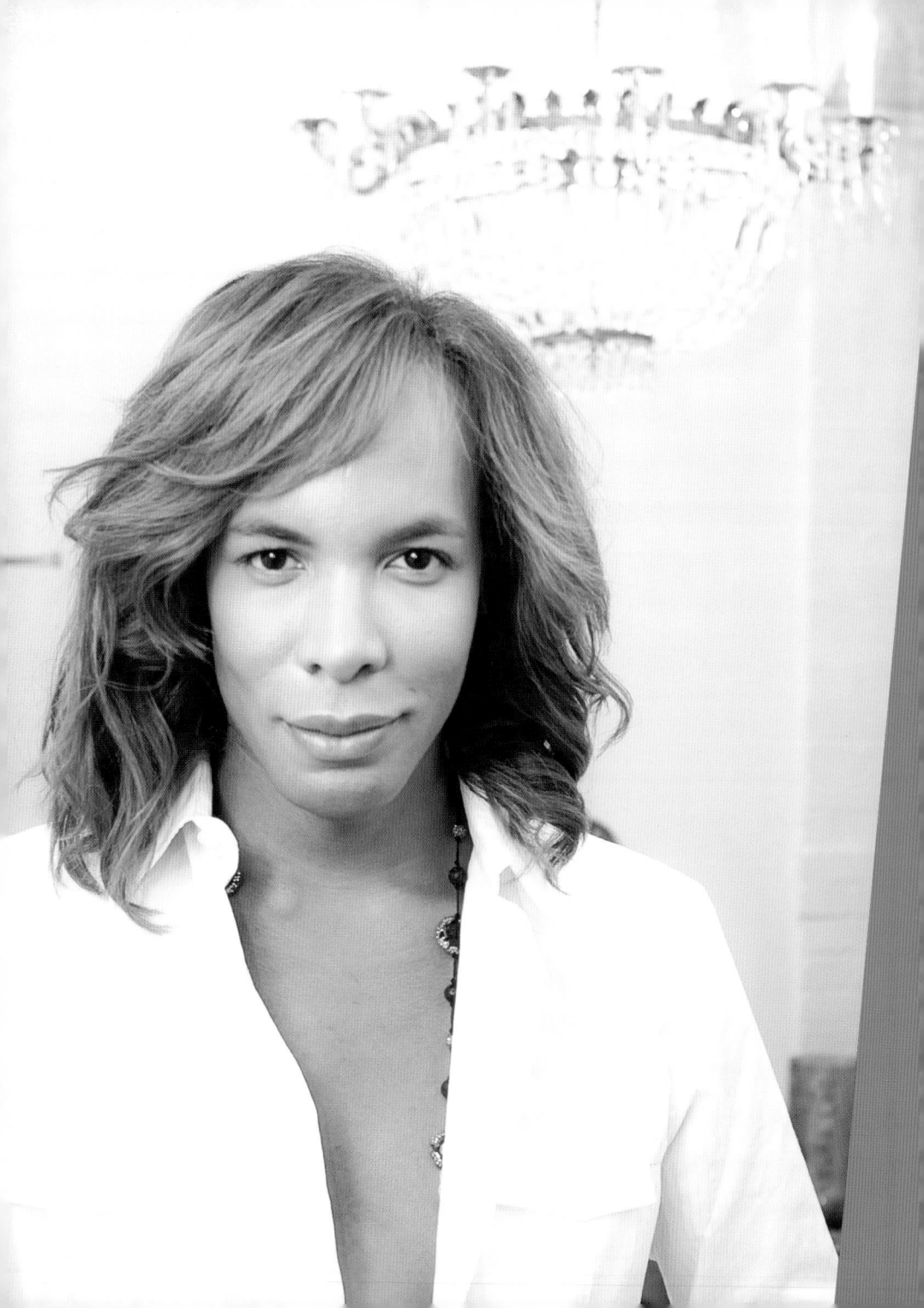

PAUL'S LAST WORD

So there it is, my simple five-step facial skincare routine (plus some advice for your body). The key to a great regimen (like everything else in this book) is to keep it simple. This is really a four-step routine for most of the week and then you switch in the exfoliation once per week—so it's even simpler than I promised!

Take the time to find the right products, set your routine, and then it's easy and you'll be able to do it in a few minutes. It will cost you no extra time to add in a toner and a rejuvenating serum, so give them a try. You now know . . .

GREAT SKIN
IS ACHIEVABLE

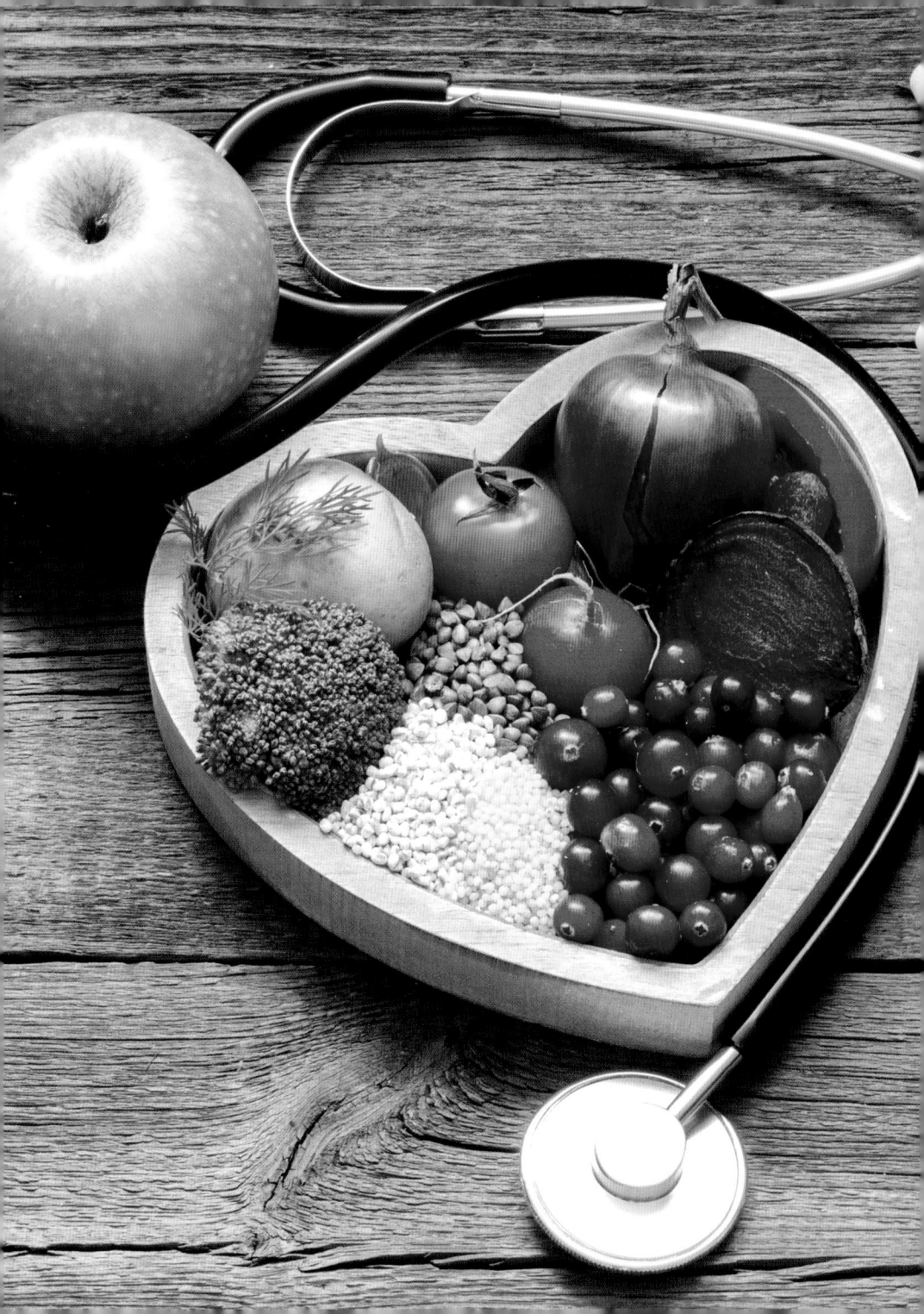

CHAPTER 4

FEEDING & BUILDING
YOUR INNER GODDESS
EAT AND DRINK WELL EVERYDAY

My family had a running joke about me needing a nap right after I ate. During the holidays, I would anticipate the big family dinners with fried chicken, baked macaroni and cheese, candied yams, and corn bread. And although I was a bit embarrassed by my reputation as a chronic napper, I couldn't help but search out a dark corner where I could secretly sleep off my food hangover.

After years of thinking that I had some form of narcolepsy, I consulted with nutritional expert and juicing guru Karliin Brooks about how I felt. I realized that the excessive fat and sugar in my food was causing my body to go through all sorts of crazy up and down changes. Karliin challenged me to a juice cleanse and designed a maintenance program to keep my energy flowing consistently throughout my busy days.

Finally, I discovered that I wasn't a chronic napper, and I could avoid crazy mood swings and emotional pitfalls by eating great quality foods and cold pressed juices. Now, I feel as youthful and energetic as I ever have before in my life and I want to share some of the things I have learned and apply myself.

THIS IS NOT A DIET

...I repeat

A quick word: I am not a personal trainer or a dietician, but I got my start in this business by instructing models at some of the world's top modeling agencies on how to achieve their best look. I've tried pretty much every form of diet known to humankind but personally, I've stayed mostly slim and in good shape due to consistency and learning how to balance. After years of working with models and making people over on TV, I know a thing or two about how to manage food, diets, and looking good.

The thing is, I LOVE food. I hosted a cooking and entertaining show a few years back. I have an appreciation for delicious cuisine from around the world and I'm not a fan of deprivation, but I do believe in moderation. So you are not going to hear me say things like "carbs are the enemy," because frankly, carbs are delicious. But so are vegetables, salads, and fruit.

Over the past fifteen years, I've worked on developing wellness programs with some of my good friends who are trainers, dieticians, and chefs, people who have set up their own juice bars and have studied how the body works.

This is not a diet because I am not telling you to lose weight. Like I said in the

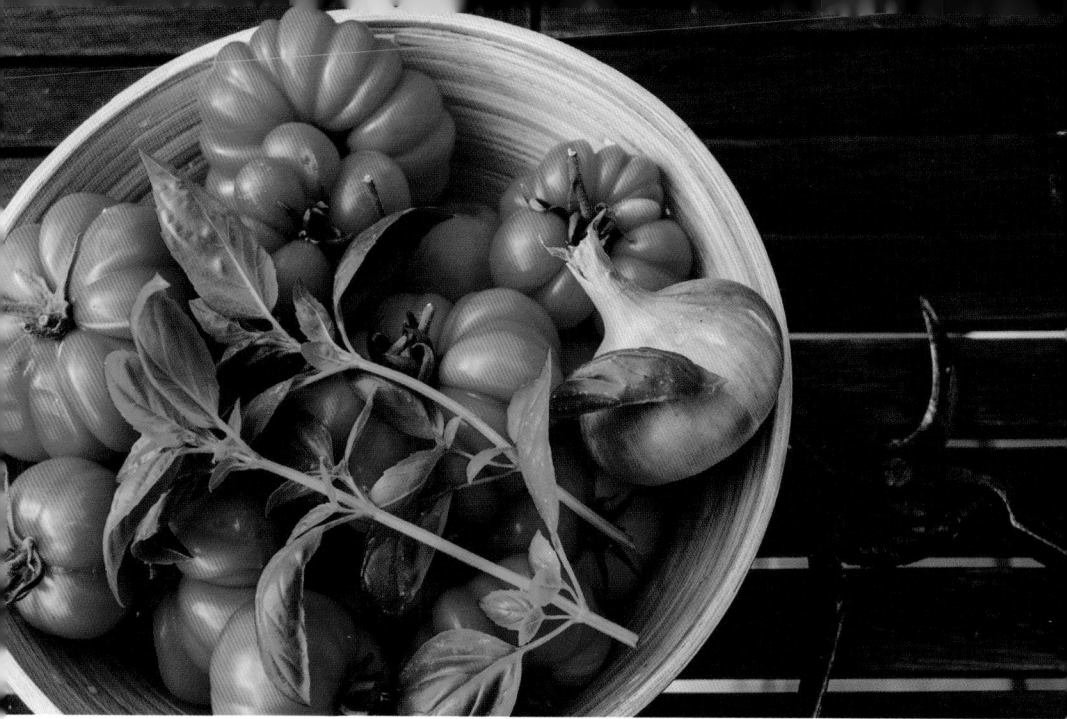

first chapter of this book—dress for the shape you are, embrace that. But, with just some small changes every day you can improve your health, energy, and happiness, plus you may drop a few pounds too.

With that disclaimer, here are some of my key tips for diet and exercise to help you feel better.

Note: Before undertaking any exercise or using the recipes or suggestions in this book, please consult a medical professional to ensure that you have no allergies, injuries, or conditions that may be exacerbated by any of these steps. These are illustrative only and may not be suitable for all people. Please diet and exercise responsibly.

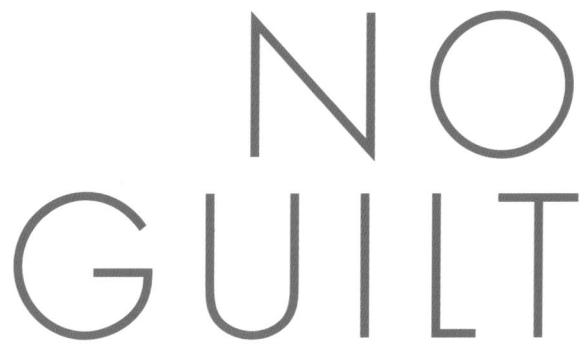

NO GUILT

How To Stay Strong Through Slips And Binges

Some people say food is just fuel. You need it to make your engine run and keep you alive. So this makes things simple: If you have a car, you need to fill up the tank when it's empty and choose the best form of fuel to make it run efficiently. Just like your body. Food is just fuel. Right?

Of course not!

Food is so much more than that. Food is emotion, it's joy, it's memories. Food triggers parts of your brain and releases hormones, food reminds you of the fondest moments in your life, food comforts you when you're sad and gets you excited when you think about it. I still remember the glorious smell of my mother's rice pudding baking in the oven when I came home from school as a boy. However, I realize that I can't eat rice pudding every day and still button my jeans! The emotional attachment to food gives it a much bigger place than it deserves in our minds and can leave us feeling trapped by it.

Here's something that I've done a hundred times: I've been eating really good, healthy food for weeks and then something really upsetting happens, it knocks me down, or I've had a crazy busy period and am just exhausted and fed up, so I turn to my go-to comfort food, fried chicken. There's nothing wrong with fried chicken–but if I were to just go nuts and order crazy amounts, eating it non-stop for several days with candied yams and macaroni and cheese, I'd have a big problem. This would send my body into overdrive–it's being hit by crazy sugar highs, bursts of fats, and artificial things that it doesn't even know how to process. My brain doesn't stand a chance, it's so busy trying to work out what the heck to do that my moods are swinging around and by the end of it I feel depressed and guilty.

Sound familiar?

Well, that's okay, it happens to all of us. It's a very natural cycle, especially if we are trying to lose some weight or keep control of our diet. The danger is that we spin into a vicious cycle where we crash and binge, feel guilty, and give food a bigger place than it deserves. If you break good habits and binge out, don't feel bad. It's okay–the next meal is like a new day and you can start fresh.

The most important advice here is not to let it own you, don't let yourself think, *oh well, I've ruined it now so I may as well give up,* or, *I can't stick to this for more than a week so it'll never work.*

DON'T BE SO HARD ON YOURSELVES.

Remember, it's just a set of chemical reactions making you feel that way. Instead, accept that you ate a bit too much and take it for what it is–just food. And the wonderful thing about food is you always get another shot–the next meal. Take a breath, don't feel guilty, and just move on by making a better choice for the next bite you take. We've all been there and we will all be there again.

YOUR BODY IS A TEMPLE

Love It With Great Food

I want you to think of your body as perfect; I don't care what shape you are, how you look, or how you used to be thinner or stronger, and so on. The simple truth is that your body is amazing, it is a beautiful thing which makes you who you are. Love it. A big mistake I have found with models and celebrities is that the spotlight and drive for a particular shape and figure means they only see their flaws. I've even heard people say that the best thing is to "hate your body" so that you punish it everyday and try to make it better.

That may work for some, but not for me. I prefer to take the opposite approach: Love your body and show it the respect that you would show to something that you love. You are taking care of it on the outside by following my advice about skin and haircare. You are showing it off by taking my tips on style. Now imagine that you are maintaining that perfect body . . . how would you treat something that you really love and respect? By giving it the very best things for it.

Every meal you have a choice: You can take an option that is bad for your body, or one that is good for it. It's that simple. If you take the bad option enough times then your body gets used to it, it expects to receive that bad choice, and so it comes to crave it. But if you start giving it good things, it will get used to that and start to crave those.

This does not mean you need to eat lettuce every meal, or cut out bread, or never eat chips. It just means that you should remember each mealtime is a choice. So choose what's better for your body, it will thank you for it and you will feel better for it.

My best advice here is preparation–we are all busy, which means we will usually pick the easiest option. This is where things get simple–just make sure the easiest option is also the best choice for your body. You will always pick it.

When you go to the grocery store try not to buy chocolate, chips, pies, and cakes unless you need them for entertaining or a special occasion. If they aren't in your pantry, then you won't eat them. Simple.

Buy vegetables instead of fries, choose peanut butter that's 100 percent peanuts without added salt, choose juice that's not from concentrate without added sugar. These things make a difference, and if you nail it in the shopping cart, then you nail it in the kitchen.

When you cook, don't fry everything, broil it. Don't add oil unless you need it, don't add butter unless you need it. Set your habits.

When you shop, when you cook, and when you eat, always remember—*I have a choice, am I making the best one for my body?*

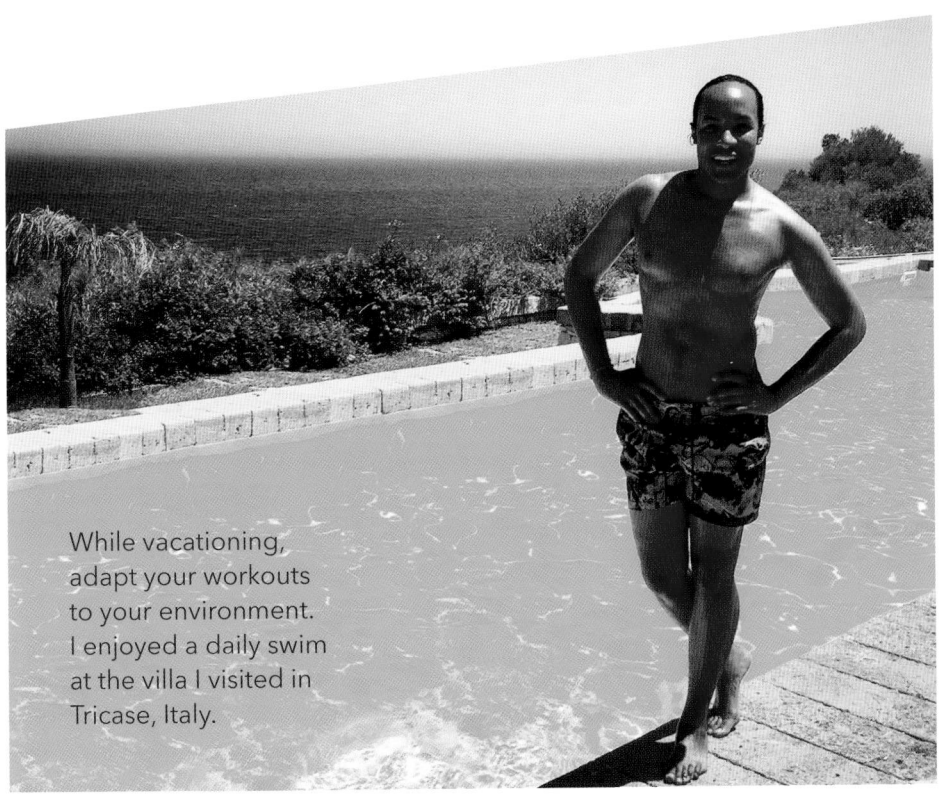

While vacationing, adapt your workouts to your environment. I enjoyed a daily swim at the villa I visited in Tricase, Italy.

ENERGIZE

PERFECT JUICES & SMOOTHIES TO POWER THROUGH EVERY DAY

Some people treat juices and smoothies like they are a crazy miracle cure for all health issues. Sadly that's not true. Remember, even juices with "no added sugar" have natural sugar; this will still give you a spike in energy and then a crash. A lot of smoothies off the shelf have additives and other ingredients which also mess with your system. Don't believe the marketing hype; just because it's a juice or a smoothie doesn't automatically mean it's the best choice for you. And they do not cancel out other choices, so don't think that a glass of OJ with your double bacon cheeseburger makes any positive difference. All you are doing there is adding a burst of sugar to your fatty meal.

That said, if you make your own or find a great local spot that makes cold pressed juices and natural smoothies the right way, they can be a great addition to your diet. I treat juices and smoothies as a way to supplement my intake of the good stuff like veggies and fruit. Here are some great and simple recipes from my friends that can help, taste great, are easy to do, and will help your body.

By the way, I haven't put specific proportions here. This is because I don't use them myself and I don't want you to be measuring everything out perfectly. Make it as quick and convenient as possible and whatever mix works for your personal taste.

Just before you start blending, I recommend you check that your machine can handle the fruit and veg in the recipes. Most will be fine so long as you chop up the items before adding them and do it in stages. I personally invested in a blender designed for smoothies which can handle all types of raw items. Do a little research and it's worth it in the long run.

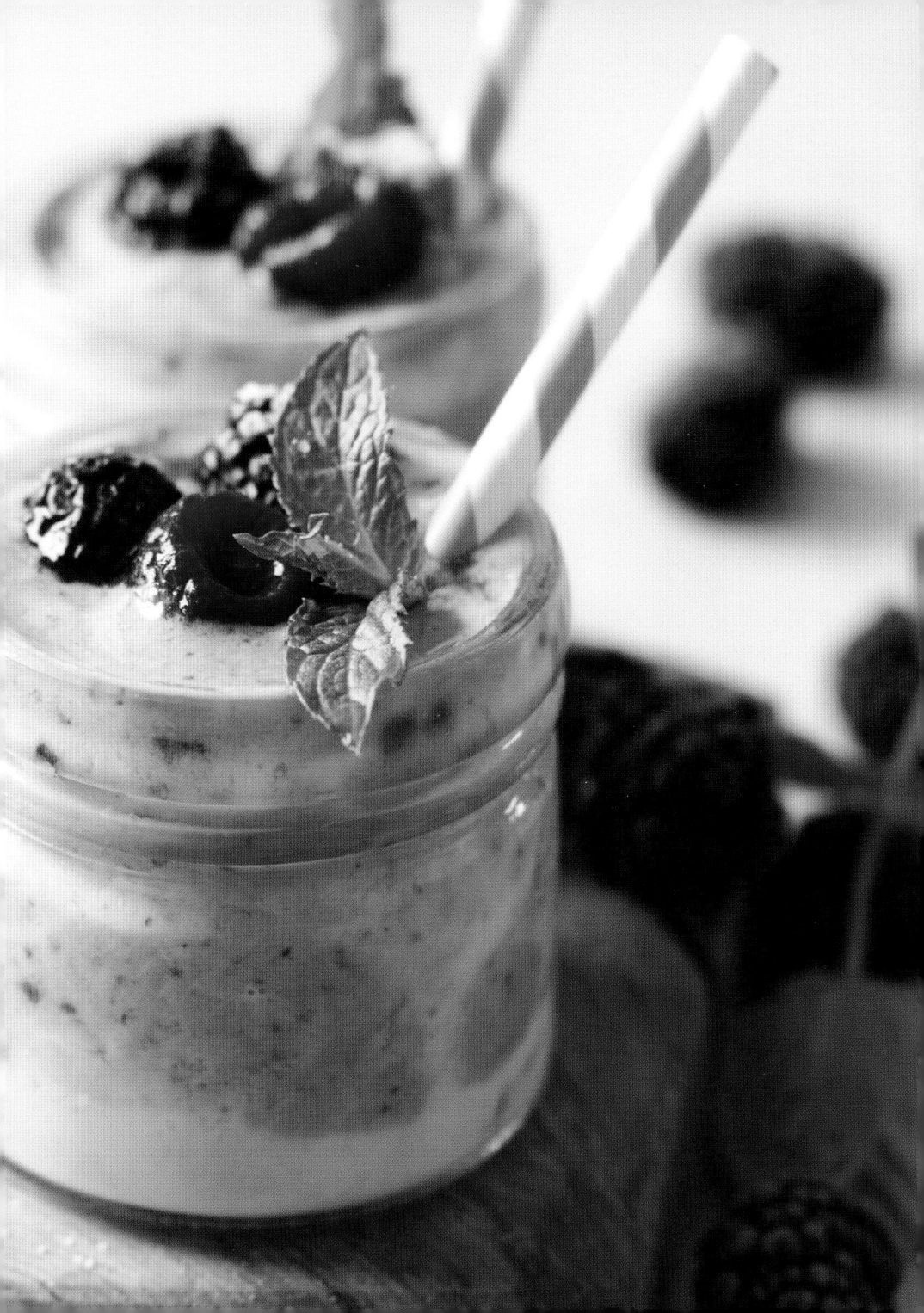

KALE, ZUCCHINI, AND BLUEBERRY WITH MANGO JUICE

I know what you're thinking: Could there be a worse drink than something with kale *and* zucchini? But try it and trust me. This is a way to get a portion of your raw veg in easily, it is a great tasting combination, and is way easier than eating a salad or portion of vegetables.

- Two good handfuls of raw kale
- Half a zucchini
- One handful of blueberries
- One glass of mango juice

Very simple—throw it all into a blender, hit the power until it's all smooth, and enjoy. The mango juice makes it sweet, the blueberries add tang and the kale and zucchini give you a great hit of vitamins.

SPINACH, AVOCADO, PEAR, AND APPLE JUICE

The avocado gives this a really smooth texture.

- Half an avocado (remove the stone and the skin)
- Two handfuls of spinach
- One pear (don't peel it, just wash it and cut off the top and bottom ends)
- One glass of apple juice

Again—just throw it all together in a blender.

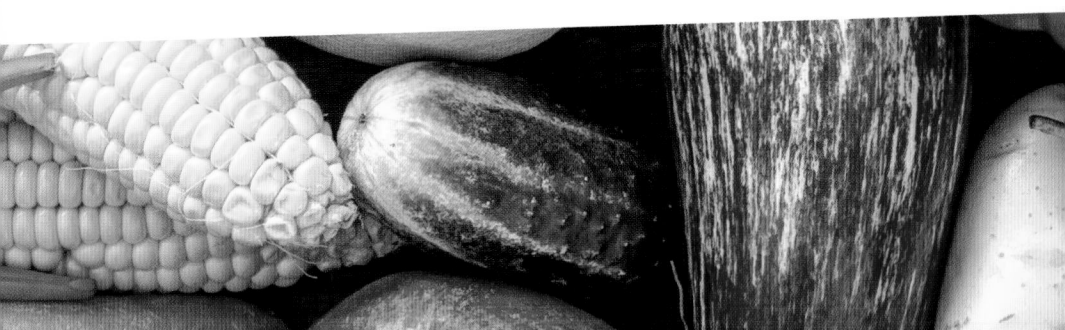

CARROT, GINGER, CELERY, AND APPLE JUICE

This is a really fresh tasting drink and my go-to daily recipe. It's also easy for me to find carrot, ginger, and apple cold-pressed juice at my local Whole Foods store.

- Two carrots (washed and peeled, cut off the top and bottom ends)
- Teaspoon of ginger (you can get fresh ginger and grate it first, or buy pre-ground ginger)
- Two sticks of celery
- Half glass of apple juice
- Ice cubes (optional)

Chop the carrots first, just to make it easier for your blender (unless you have a very powerful blender).

Paul's Expert Tip

If you want to be adventurous, add a kick of spice by putting a quarter of a teaspoon of cayenne pepper, or a quarter of a chopped chili pepper. You don't need much, but it's a perfect way to wake up in the morning.

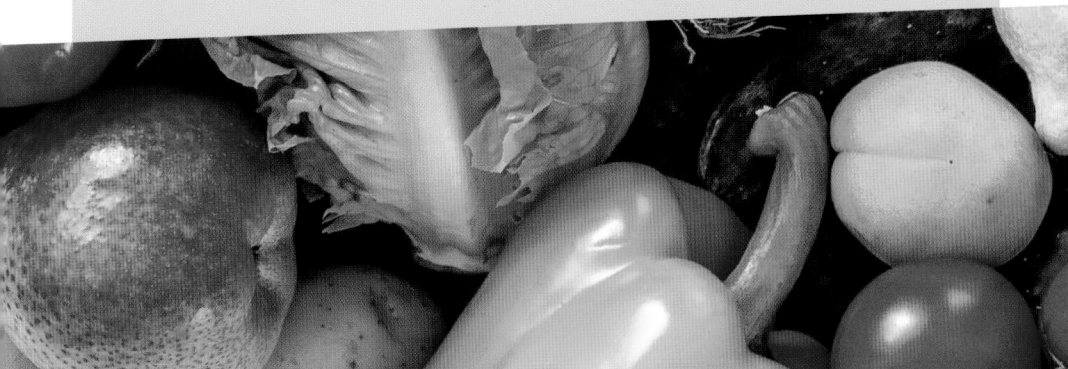

FIVE
EASY CHANGES
THAT WILL MAKE YOU FEEL AMAZING

1 Eating out—if you're at a restaurant, swap out the carbs (whether they are fries, bread, rice, or anything else) for a side of vegetables. This doesn't have to be a plain side salad—ask them what they can do and pick something tasty. It's an easy way to get a little more veg into your day.

2 Pick the salad—it's a regular lunchtime choice; you can get a salad or a sandwich. My advice is to take the salad. I have my own go-to salad spot called Sweetgreen that makes my salads about five days a week. They know just the way I like it and there's a lot of tasty options so I can switch it up from time to time. Sounds obvious, but it's hard to do. So make the decision ahead of time—know that you are going to choose a salad in advance and always choose one that will taste good and fill you up.

3 Skip the sugar—you're run down, tired, in need of something to pick you up in the middle of the day and you go for that candy bar . . . stop. That chocolate is not going to help you. You'll get a spike of sugar that throws your concentration off and then a crash that leaves you feeling low AND it won't fill you up. Go for something else. If there is a protein option like almonds, take that (protein options make you feel full for longer), otherwise some veggie sticks or a piece of fruit.

I'm keeping this short and simple. There are a thousand changes I could suggest, but as with everything in this book I want you to take sustainable steps and be realistic. So here are just five easy changes; make these adjustments and I believe you will notice the difference. They are achievable and manageable no matter how hectic your life may be.

By the way, this includes protein and granola bars. Those things will sit in your stomach, often have a lot of sugar and additives, and are not a healthy alternative. If you want protein, the best thing is to get some nuts, a hard-boiled egg, tuna fish (I prefer the Chunk Light Tongol Tuna from Whole Foods) or something else natural.

4 Stick to water—I shouldn't need to tell you that fizzy sodas are bad for you, but sugar-free versions can be just as bad. Fruit juices are fine in moderation but they still have sugar. Water keeps you hydrated, it helps your skin, your brain, and best of all it's usually free! I suggest adding lemon to your water. Lemons are an ionic, which makes the water alkaline as your body digests it. You will hydrate more efficiently when drinking alkaline water.

5 Cut out one sugary item from your daily diet—Why am I emphasizing sugar so much? Because sugar impacts your concentration and moods, it affects your body in many ways and above all else, it's almost addictive. The more you eat, the more you want. Your taste buds get used to it and need bigger and stronger amounts otherwise you don't feel satisfied. Here's the good news: If you can cut back on your sugar little by little, you need less of it. Your taste buds will adapt the other way, and eventually you will find some things too sweet.

WHETHER IT IS SKIPPING SUGAR

in your tea or coffee, dropping one candy bar each day, or swapping out a soda for water.

THIS SIMPLEST OF CHANGES

will have an effect and make you want less and less.

Although high in natural sugar, red wine is full of healthy antioxidants—at least that's my excuse!

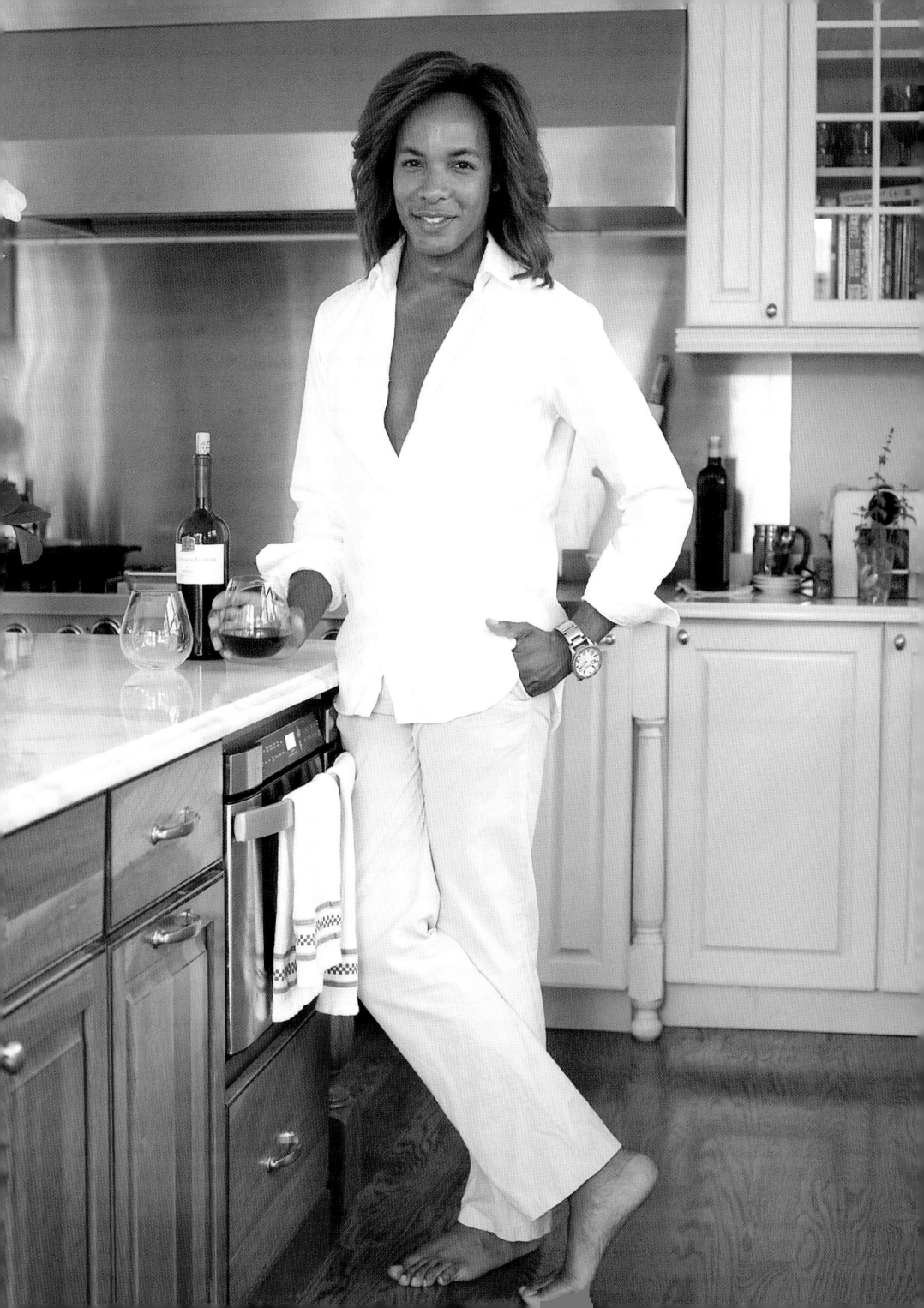

EXERCISE
IS NOT PUNISHMENT
Learn How to Enjoy Working Out

I have never been a natural athlete. I was never a track star or the first pick on the James H. Harrison Elementary School kickball team, I didn't do gymnastics, and while I do enjoy watching a good NBA game, I was never more than average at playing basketball. So, exercise doesn't come naturally to me. I would rather spend an hour of my free time hanging out with my friends, visiting my family, even just watching Netflix or listening to my favorite Spotify playlist than exercising. That is, I used to be like that. After trying all kinds of workouts from high intensity interval training, to spin classes, weights, yoga, and some crazy fad that I prefer to forget, I realized that my workouts went in cycles.

I would go through a period where I worked out all the time, then I'd slip off, lose my rhythm, and struggle. I started looking at the periods where I had real discipline and realized that it wasn't discipline, it was pleasure. I had done lots of exercise because I was really enjoying the exercise at that time.

So here are my two pieces of advice.

MAKE IT FUN

Find something that you actually enjoy and makes you feel good; back in my parents' day, the options were limited to Jane Fonda videos (if you remember those), sweating to the oldies with Richard Simmons (I miss you Richard!), or embarrassing yourself in a class full of people who all looked super serious and focused. Those days are gone. We now have a wider than ever variety of options. So try everything you can, don't just join a gym and walk on a treadmill until you get bored and go home. Don't be afraid to enter the free weights area just because there are a bunch of guys there grunting while they lift their own bodyweight. Try every class you can, try every form you can, and find what makes you buzz. Forget about how you look when you start—nobody is perfect the first time. There was a time when Michael Phelps couldn't swim, when Usain Bolt wasn't very fast. Everybody starts somewhere.

A friend of mine recently told me they had really gotten into spin classes, more specifically Soul Cycle. This person had expected to hate it, they'd tried it years ago and it didn't work for them, but they were convinced to try a different studio and they loved it. So much that they go several times a week and look forward to it. If they hadn't tried that first class then they would have continued treating exercise like a box they have to check each day to feel worthwhile.

MAKE IT EASY

I don't mean the exercise itself—I mean make it accessible. The easier you make it for you to work out, the more likely you are to enjoy it and keep doing it. This involves simple choices: pick a gym close to your home or work, choose exercise classes that are on your way home, find somewhere with nice people who are supportive and upbeat.

There are many ways to make it easy, but what you want is to set up exercise so you can comfortably fit it into your day and ensure that it's in a place with people that you are happy to be around.

THE CORE OF IT ALL

Simple Exercises That Will Improve Your Life

I am generally not giving you specific exercise advice, but here is one area that I believe is so important that I wanted to give you something to actually do. Nearly all of us neglect our core and most misunderstand it. But it's one of the easiest things to fix and will give you some of the biggest benefits in life.

Firstly, I'm not just talking about your abs and I don't even care about you having a six-pack. We all know about our abdominal muscles that sit underneath the layer of skin and fat at the front of our bodies. But think of the core as being a corset that extends all the way around your body including your sides and your back. It is like a support structure that holds you up and keeps you balanced. Take care of your core and it will take care of you in return.

Paul's Expert Tip

Get a support system. It's much easier and more fun to work out when you have people with you, whether it's having your other half take care of the kids or sort out dinner so you can fit in a class, or joining a gym with some friends (you might even get a referral bonus).

The beauty of the core is that you only need to spend a few minutes to make a big difference. But remember, don't worry about how it looks on the outside, it's all about what's underneath. If you starve yourself for long enough and then get dehydrated, you will eventually have a six-pack, but that doesn't mean your core will be strong. You can do these three exercises in less than five minutes (you can make them go a lot longer if you want, of course—this is just for starters), so try setting your alarm five minutes earlier and doing them every day for two weeks. You will feel a difference.

Before doing any of these, please consult with a doctor and make sure it is safe to do so. If you experience discomfort then stop immediately.

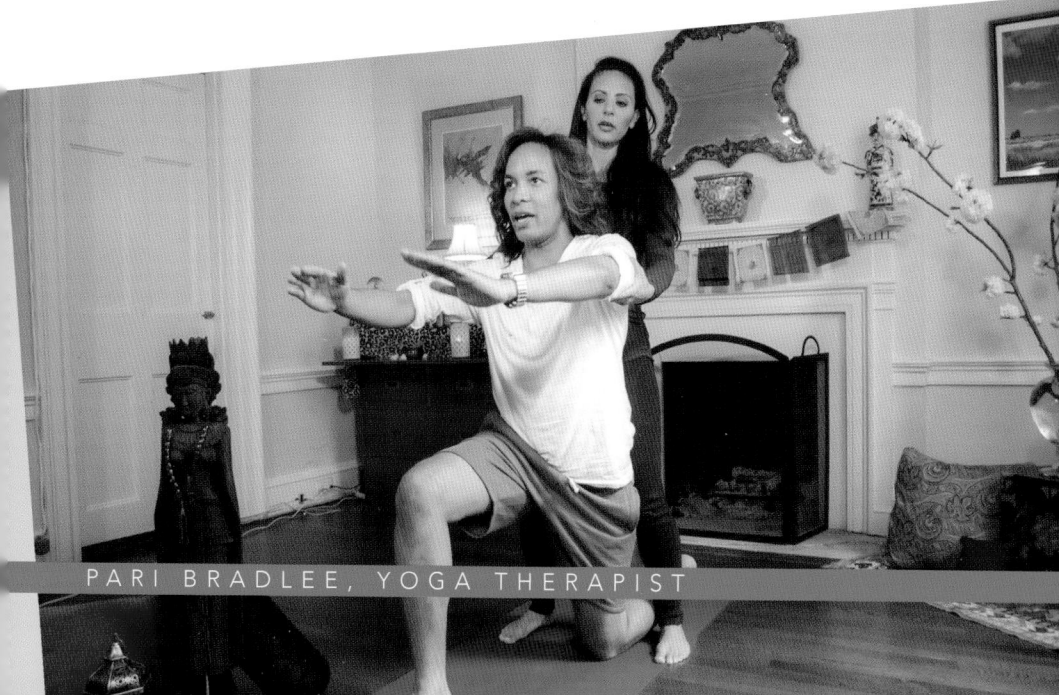

PARI BRADLEE, YOGA THERAPIST

THE PLANK / THE SUPERMAN

One of the best exercises ever, it is low impact and you can modify it to be easier in the beginning and harder as you get better. Start with this to warm up your core.

There's a bunch of names for this exercise but I like the whole superhero idea so I stuck with this one. It works your back, and again, you can modify it to make it easy or harder.

Lie face-down on the floor with your legs shoulder-width apart and your arms lying palm-down in front of your body. Slowly raise your arms and legs off the ground at the same time, then hold them up for a few seconds and then lower in a slow and controlled fashion before repeating.

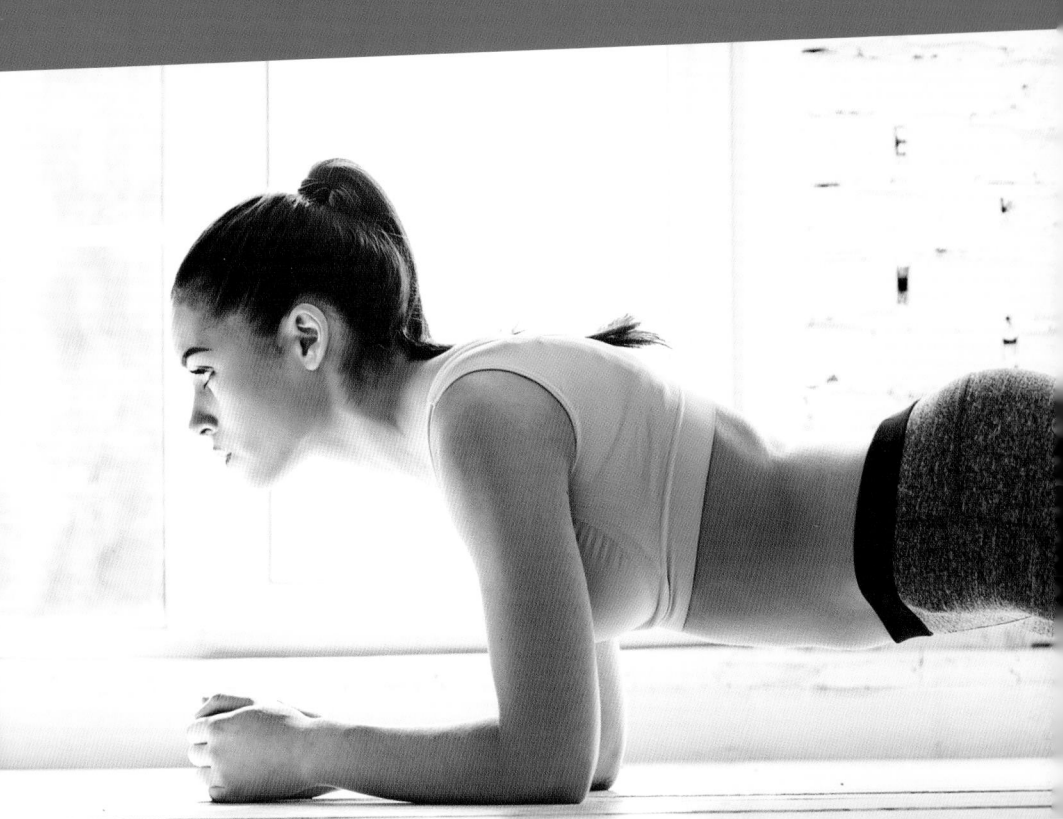

ABDOMINAL CRUNCHES

Don't confuse these with "sit-ups." I just want you to come up part of the way and really focus on tightening those abs as you do it. Work the lower part of your core and be careful not to pull your lower back.

SQUATS

Finish with these, and really focus on the stance and technique as you can see below. There's a right way to do squats and a lot of people get it wrong, but once you've warmed up the core, bust out as many of these as you can. No weights needed. Take them slowly if you are new—the best thing is to do them safely and gently in the beginning until you get comfortable.

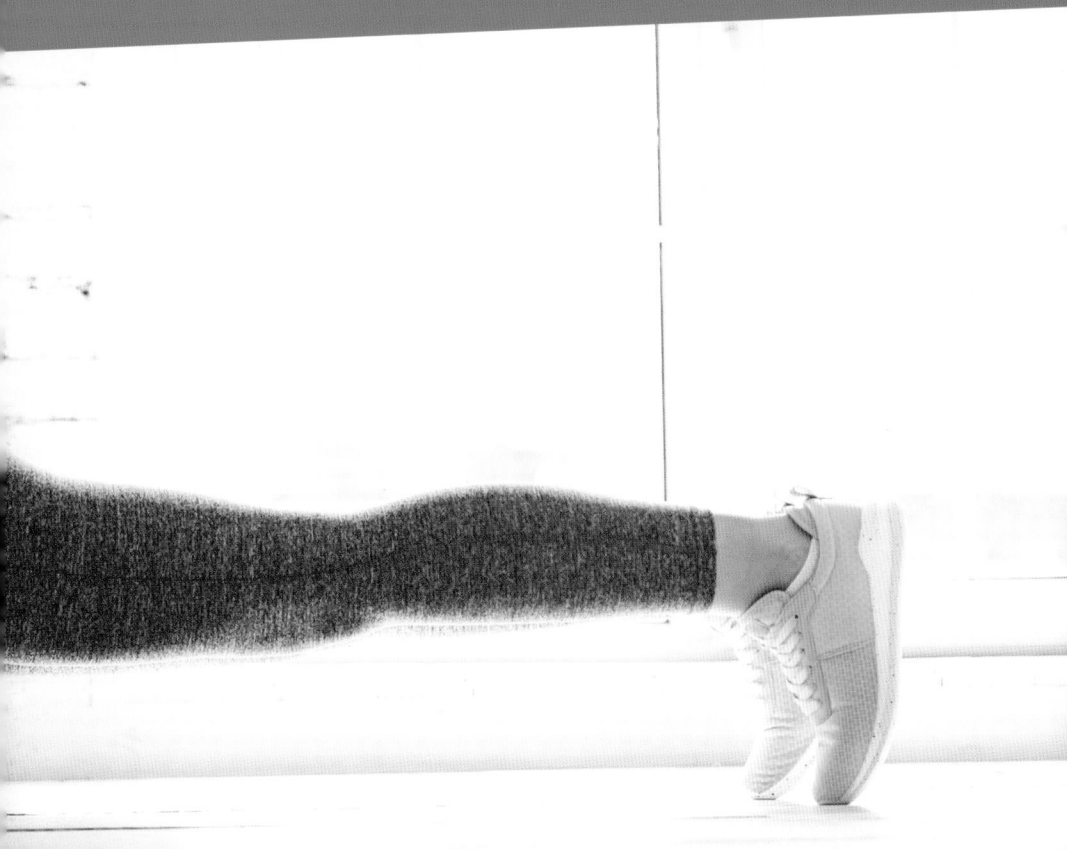

SWEAT IT OUT

How to Fit in Cardio on a Tight Schedule

I'm going to bust an old myth—longer workouts aren't automatically better than shorter workouts. In the old days, we used to think you had to run for two hours straight to burn calories effectively. Fortunately, now we know better and efficiency is key. You can get on a treadmill or bike for an hour and have a less effective workout than spending fifteen minutes jumping rope. It's all about how you spend your time.

The type of cardio that best suits you will depend on your own body and what you can handle. But if you haven't exercised for a while, that's not a bad thing—it means you will get gains very quickly at the beginning. Don't set yourself impossible targets—start small and build up the difficulty.

A very effective way to do this is with HIIT, aka High Intensity Interval Training. This term can cover a whole range of things so don't be put off by it or think there is only one way to make it work. You can apply the basic principle to any form of cardio and it will help you get the most out of your time. The idea is to set intervals for sprinting and recovering. For example, if you normally do thirty minutes on an exercise bike, instead of going at a steady pace the whole time, try doing a five-minute warm-up and then sprint for one minute and take a steady (not slow) pace for thirty seconds, and keep repeating this approach.

You will burn more calories than cycling for thirty minutes at the same speed.

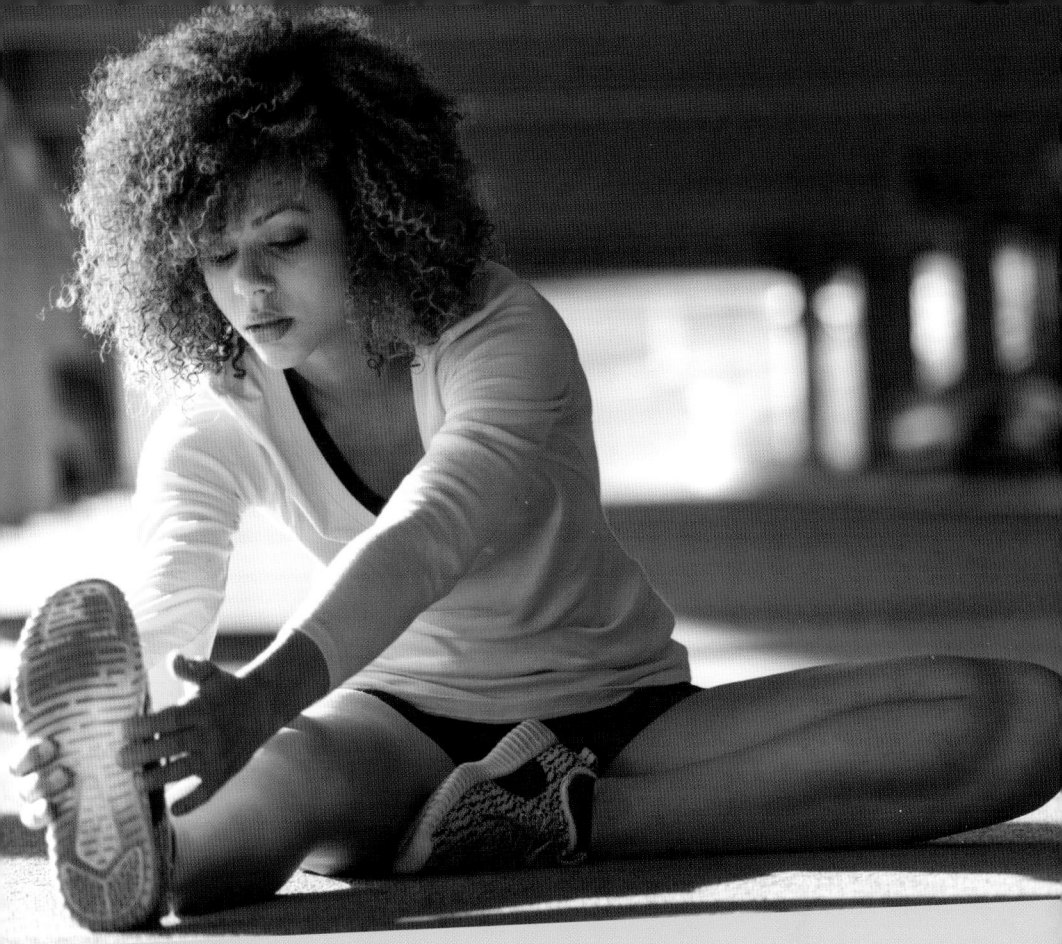

Paul's Expert Tip

If you go running, it's really easy to do HIIT. As a kid, I had asthma and I thought that meant that I could never be a runner. In fact, I spent most of my twenties and now my thirties telling my trainers that I couldn't run. But one day, I got on the treadmill and did a mile, and then two, three miles became four, and that became six. After telling myself for most of my life that I couldn't run, I discovered that with an open mind and giving it a shot, I am actually a runner. The key is to keep your heart rate up. If you are jogging, try sprinting to a street corner or landmark, then jogging steadily to the next, then sprinting, and so on.

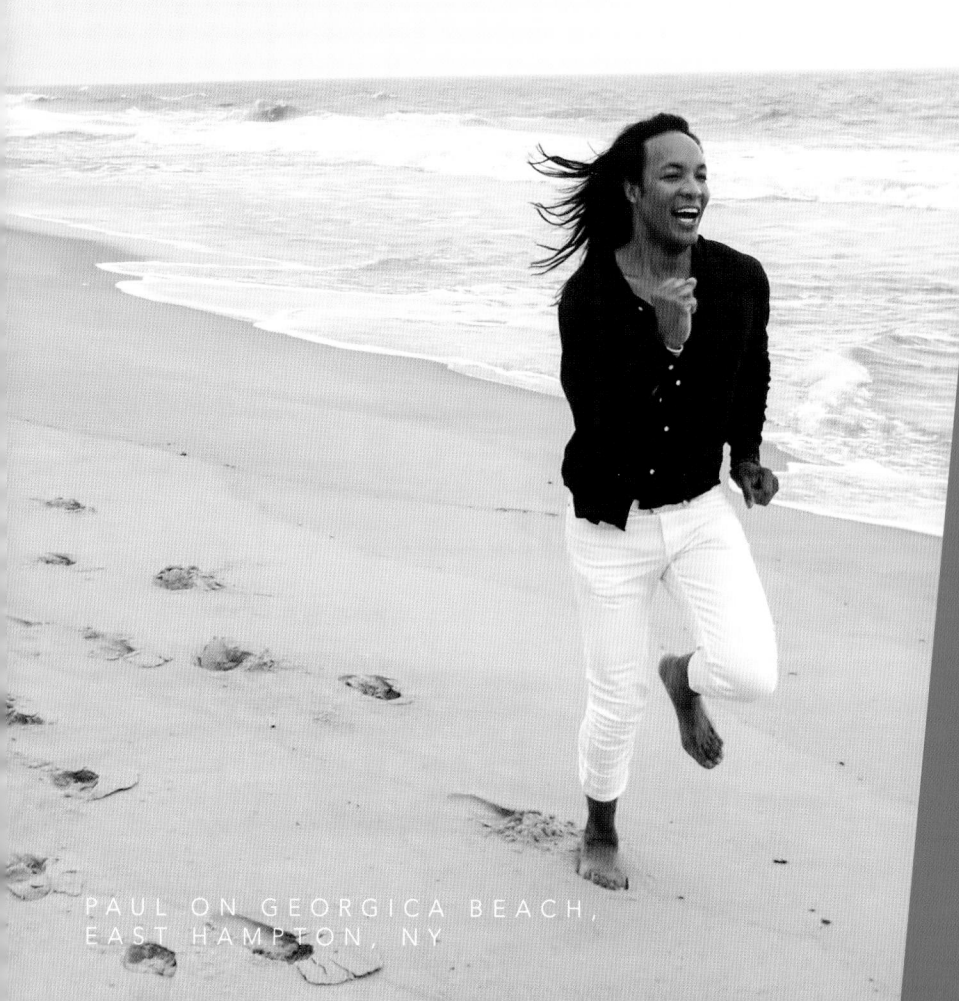

PAUL ON GEORGICA BEACH,
EAST HAMPTON, NY

PAUL'S LAST WORD

Achieving what you consider to be the most impossibly perfect body is not something I suggest you focus your energy on. There are many life experiences and downright extraordinary adventures that could be missed along the way to achieving your six-pack abs. Deciding what balance feels good for you is a personal thing and your decision to make. But I will tell you this: If you incorporate some of the tips that I've shared here, you will feel more balanced overall, your clothes will fit better, and people will generally enjoy being around you more. What you eat doesn't just affect your body, it affects your mindset, your productivity, and your relationships with others. Get going on this and . . .

WATCH YOUR BODY'S
GRATITUDE
POSITIVELY AFFECT YOUR
ATTITUDE

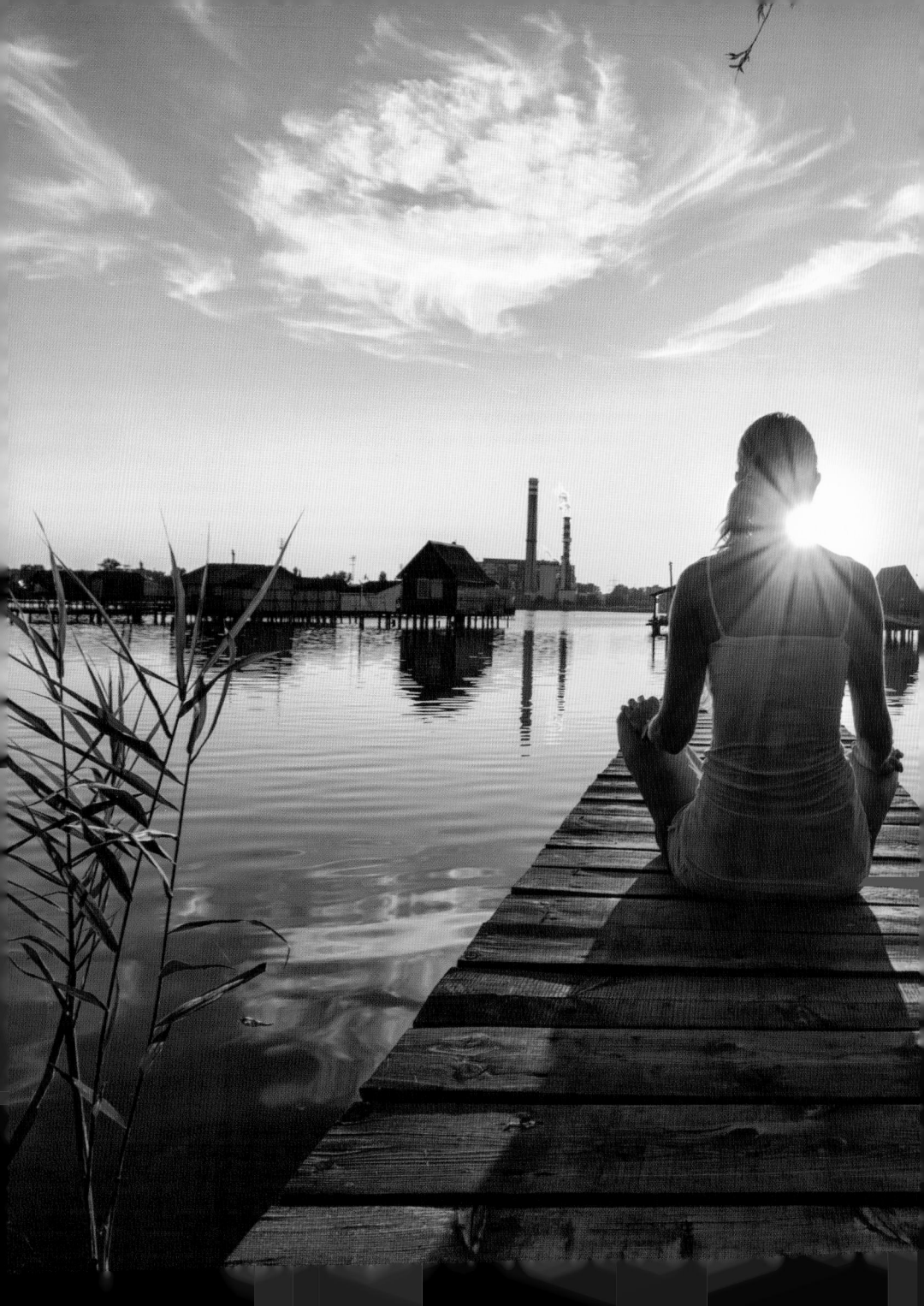

CHAPTER 5

A STRONG WOMAN

NEEDS A STRONG MIND

The first live television gig I had years ago almost caused me to pass out cold. I literally had so much going on in my head at once that the room started spinning and I couldn't feel my feet below me, all happening on live TV!

I realized immediately that if I was going to have a successful career in front of the camera I would have to learn to declutter my mind and quiet random thoughts from taking over that very valuable cranial real estate! I started meditating and practicing various ways to zone in to the topic at hand.

Over the years, the noise in my head has calmed and I can now control the thoughts that I choose to focus on without feeling overwhelmed. Some of these strategies and techniques that I have been taught changed my life and I think they could do the same for you.

MIND MATTERS

So far, I have taken you through the physical layers from what you should wear (and how to wear it) to your body and how to take care of yourself in an achievable and consistent manner.

Now I want to take a little time just to focus on your mind—this is probably the most important key to being happy and if you get this right, it will help you fully pull it all together. There are many books, apps, and guides to meditation and mindfulness—I know because I've read most of them! Throughout my journey exploring mindful living, I've learned a few techniques and ways to look at life that really make a difference to me and I wanted to share them with you. Think of this chapter as Paul's personal guide to what helps him remain calm, happy, and in control. Use it as guidance and take from it whatever feels right for your life. Like the tips that I've shared in previous chapters, each person is different and I want you to find the right path for you (whether that's style, hair, makeup, or your mind).

We live in an amazing time with technology, entertainment, and opportunities that have never existed before, but this also means that our brains are bombarded with so many distractions, images, and ideas, that it is easy to lose ourselves. I know this personally; over my career, I have found myself chasing things that were no good for me just because I thought they would make me happy, and although it has taken me some time, I have learned one thing—the only way

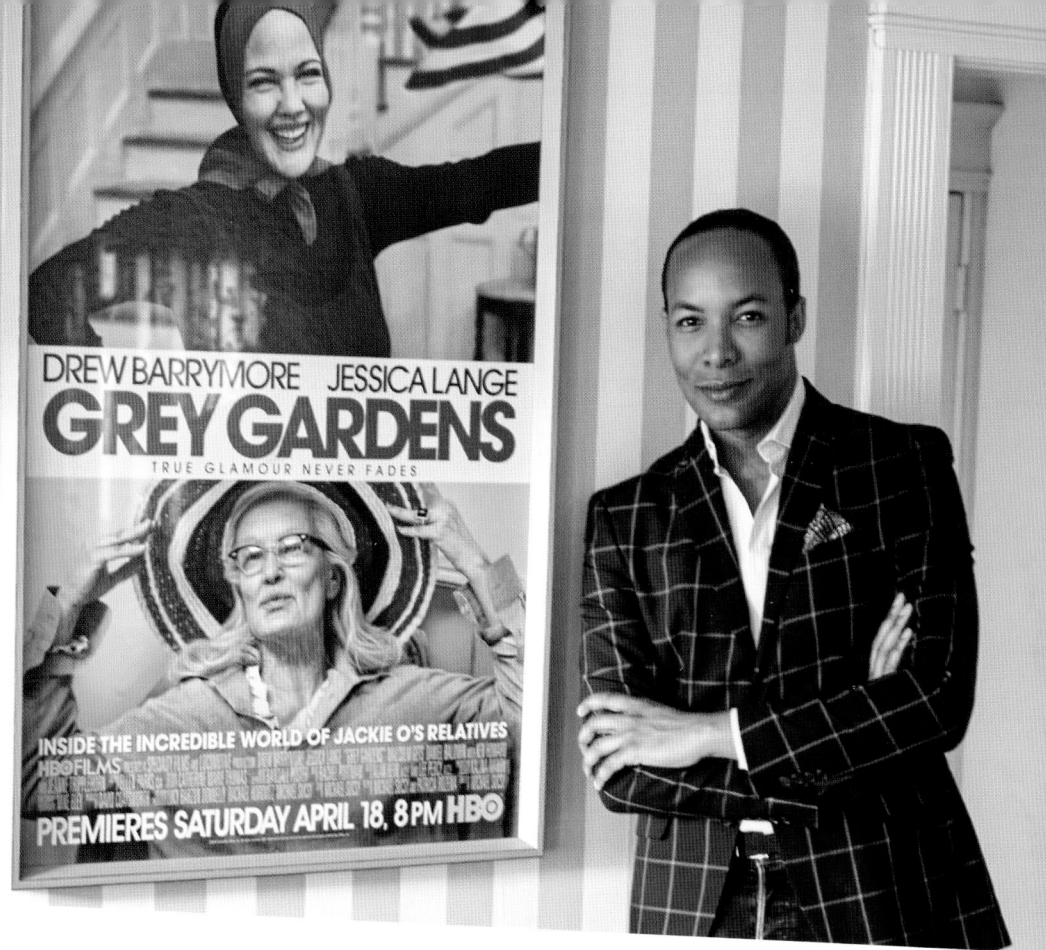

to truly be happy is to be happy in yourself. There has never been a designer bag, expensive German automobile, or Rolex watch that has ever made me feel fulfilled.

It's an easy line to throw out, harder to achieve, but I am going to give you some advice and exercises that you can do every day to help center and focus yourself. Think about it like this: you have just read and (I hope) implemented advice for the external things. Treat your mind as if it is something you want to develop and train, just a few minutes first thing in the morning and last thing at night can make a big difference.

LIVE WITHOUT CRUTCHES
You Don't Need Validation From Others

This may sound like I am telling you to cut off ties with people around you; that is usually not the case although an occasional edit of your contacts list is usually not a bad idea. You will have wonderful people who love and cherish you for the unique person that you are and you should keep those people close.

But, there is an easy mistake that we have all made in our lives at one time or another—we view ourselves through someone else's eyes. When we were young, many of us craved the approval of our parents—it's only natural. When they said they were proud of us, we felt proud of ourselves. When they were disappointed in us, we felt as if we let ourselves down.

This continues for nearly everybody, whether it is a friend, spouse, partner, colleague, or family member, there are always those people whose approval we crave. While this is quite normal, the problem comes when we get too reliant on that, because people and relationships change. If I have a friend and my confidence comes from knowing that they think I'm a good person, then what happens if we have a falling out, or we drift apart like so many people do? I am going to be lost because the person who gives me my confidence has gone away.

But what if I know deep down that I am a good person, for all my flaws I am a decent human being who deserves to be loved and to receive good things? If I fall out with my friend or we drift apart, I will be sad and disappointed, but I'm not going to question myself and whether I'm broken or not good enough.

This is not easy to achieve and we all have to work at it. For now, I just want you to think about yourself. I want you to take two minutes, sit up straight, close your eyes, take a deep breath in and out. And just remember that you are an amazing person who deserves respect and good things. I want you to think positive thoughts about yourself for just two minutes.

Do this every day when you have a quiet two minutes in your office, room, or on the train—just take two minutes to beathe and focus on your own energy.

IT'S THE END OF THE WORLD AS WE KNOW IT . . . OR NOT

Have you ever found yourself spiralling down? You made a mistake, forgot to do something, or did something completely wrong and everything seems to be falling apart. Maybe your boss was mad, your kids were upset, your partner stormed out, and you're blaming yourself. But instead of just getting upset about the mistake or the thing that went wrong, you go further and start thinking that you're useless, remembering all the other mistakes you made, times you were humiliated, maybe you even start thinking that you're not worth anything and once people realize that then you will be left alone.

This is called "catastrophizing." It's a long word that just refers to how we spiral down. This is very common, we all do it. We feel vulnerable and all our insecurities just join hands in a giant chain that looks like it will go on forever. The reason we do this is because we prioritise things right now in our lives—whatever our goal is today must be the most important thing.

I once had a clothing disaster before going on a special edition of the live television morning show that I work on. I decided to wear my crisp white shirt and tie along with my three-piece suit to the station in an attempt to save time. I worked non-stop to put everything together, I had barely slept for three nights just trying to get it all perfect and make sure no detail was missed and it looked great on the show. I was driving to the television station and when I reached for my coffee, the lid came off and it spilled on my shirt and tie. It was too late for me to do anything, I didn't have time to go home and change. I freaked out, I had this panic where I suddenly knew that the show would be a disaster, I felt in over my head, and that somehow despite all the work that I had done over the years, this would be the moment that sunk my career. I was obviously having a major melt down moment and then I remembered times that I had felt like a failure or been embarrassed and I wanted to quit and run away in the past.

In fact, I spent a few minutes panicking and then took a deep breath and calmly pulled into the station parking lot. I decided to take a look in my trunk and see if I had any spare clothing items. I found my go-to outfit, a simple white v-neck T-shirt and a pair of jeans. I grabbed the both of those and ran into the dressing room. Without consulting anyone else on the show, I showed up on set wearing the T-shirt, jeans, and the blazer from my suit, an outfit that I thought was inappropriate based on what other guys wore on the show (they all wore suits and ties). I launched my new segment with major confidence and personality and after the show the Executive Producer called me to his office. I thought he going to say that the station had a policy on men wearing ties on the show. Instead, he told me that the segment got great feedback and suggested I dressed in this relaxed style more often. I thought that without my suit and tie I would be perceived poorly and disappoint the bosses. But when I was forced to be my most authentic self and stood in my truth and confidence it ended up being a major turning point in my work at that station. I was bigger than the clothes, and my authentic personality and confidence won out in the end.

When I say it now, the idea that spilling coffee on my shirt could have seemed like such a big deal is embarrassing, but it wasn't the shirt itself, it was all my anxiety, stress, and nerves that had built up until something triggered them and they all held hands to form that chain of misery.

So how do you beat this when it happens?

THE ANSWER IS ACTUALLY SIMPLE—
YOU STOP IT.

Learn to sense when you are spiraling, when this chain of doubts is forming. Recognize that you are starting to do it, focus your mind, and say "no." Step into a separate room or the bathroom, take a few deep and slow breaths and just force your mind to stop adding to that chain. Focus on how to fix the situation, and if it can't be fixed, just try to let it go. It really won't be the end of the world, it won't even be the end of your life.

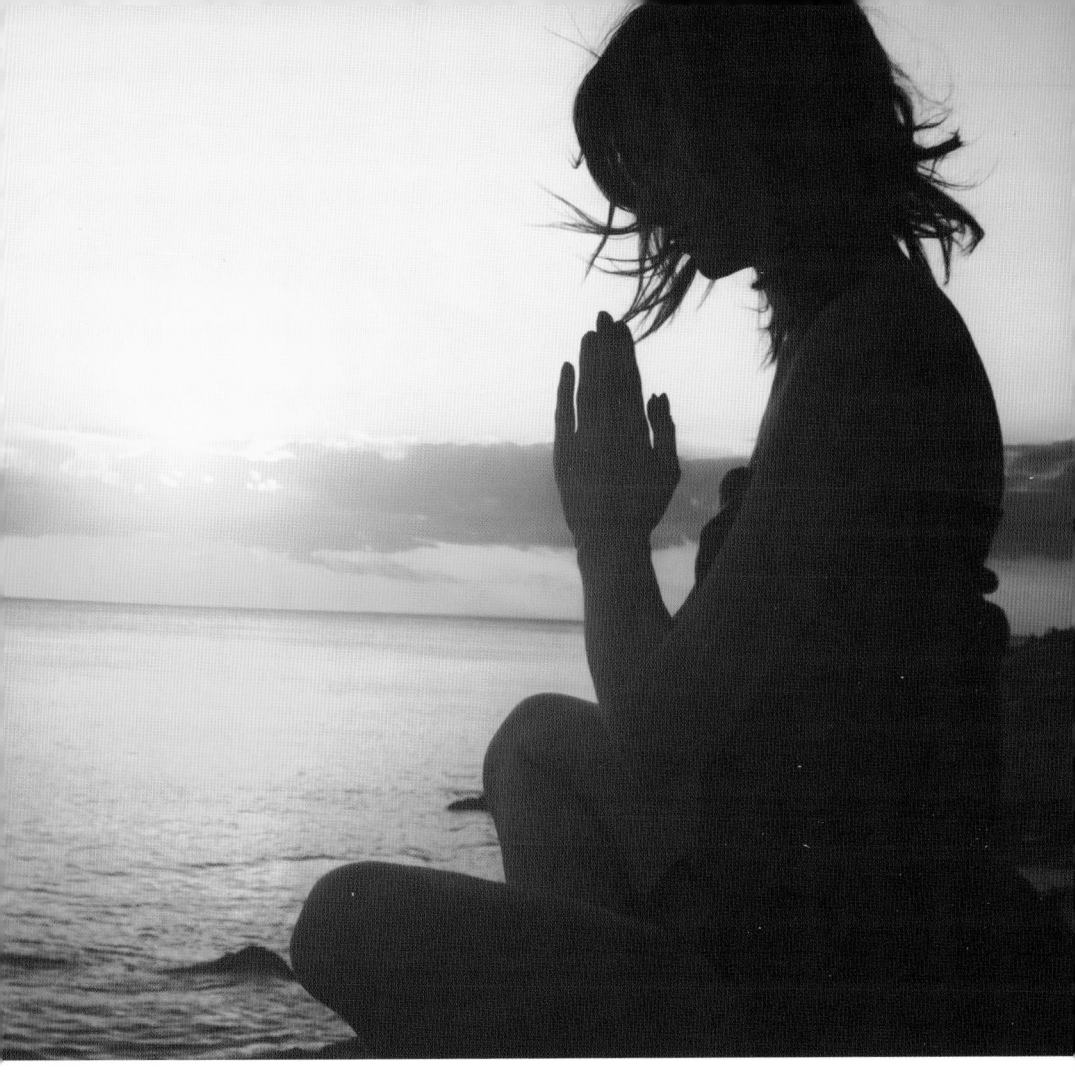

One of the best pieces of advice I ever heard was this—when you feel low, sit or stand up straight, take a deep breath in, and smile. Try it right now. When you are standing tall and smiling, it's very hard to feel sad. Maybe it is forced, but trust me, this works. Give yourself a few moments to stop the spiral, and you can then focus on making things better and moving on.

WAKE UP
ON THE RIGHT SIDE
Simple Exercises to Start Each Day the Right Way

I've read lots of motivational advice that starts with phrases like, "Treat each day as if it were your last," "Attack each day," "Life isn't a dress rehearsal so always give it 110 percent."

I don't know about you, but if I waged war on every day and performed at 110 percent all the time, I'd be so tired that I'd just go back to bed (not to mention, how the heck does someone give "10 percent" anyway?!). If you always give that much, will there be anything left?

There is one slogan that I do believe: "Life isn't a sprint, it's a marathon."

Of course sad things happen and things get cut short, but the truth is we need to find a balance to stay in the moment but still plan ahead. This is true of life in general as it is of each day. We live hectic lives, whether you have a family, job, school, or whatever, there is a stack full of pressures and things pulling your time.

So I want you to take two minutes every single morning just for yourself. And I know you're busy, but we can all spare two minutes. I do this each day. As soon as that alarm goes off, instead of sighing with a sense of dread and thinking about how little sleep you actually got and how much stuff you have to do—lie flat on your back with your arms to your side or resting on your stomach (whatever is comfortable), and close your eyes.

Do not fall back to sleep! But instead take a really big, deep breath through your nose, really fill your lungs slowly, and then slowly exhale through mouth. Do this twice, and imagine that you are slowing the world down, as if you are putting the room and everyone around you on slow motion. Focus on that feeling.

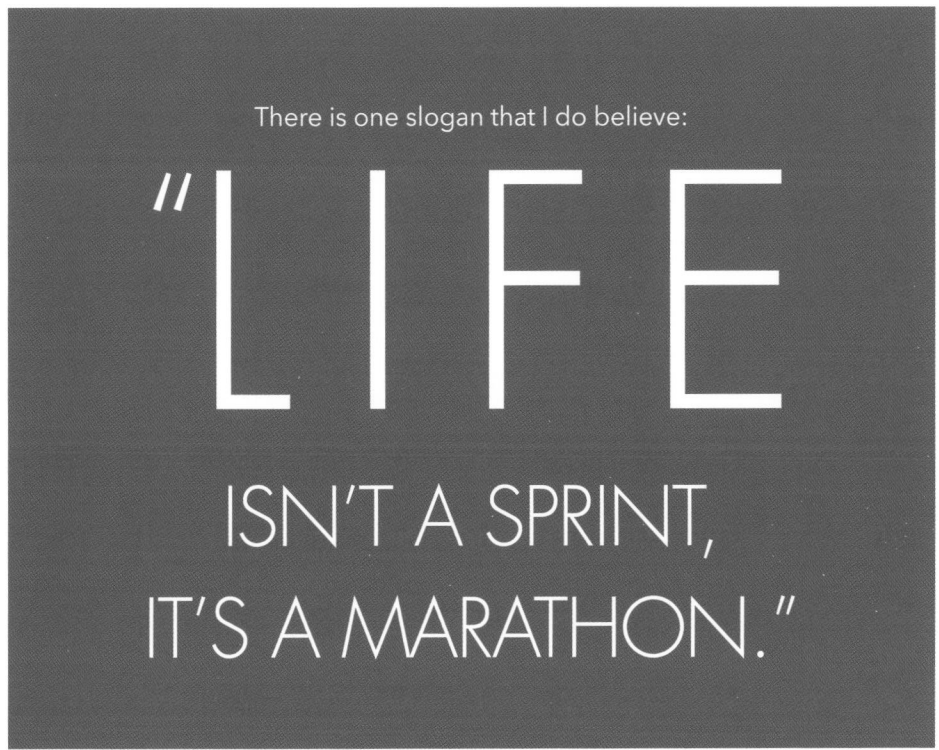

There is one slogan that I do believe:

"LIFE
ISN'T A SPRINT,
IT'S A MARATHON."

Breathe normally but keep your eyes closed and visualize the day ahead, think of it as if you are playing a video and it's on fast forward, and you are moving quickly through the day and stopping when you get to something important. For each activity you go through, visualize it as a success. I don't care if this is dropping the kids to school, driving to work and parking, having a business meeting—just see it happening smoothly and flawlessly. Take it all the way to night and see yourself getting into bed after a great successful day.

Take a final deep breath in through your nose and out through your mouth, and slowly open your eyes.

It takes only two minutes—but you will feel more relaxed and positive about the day ahead.

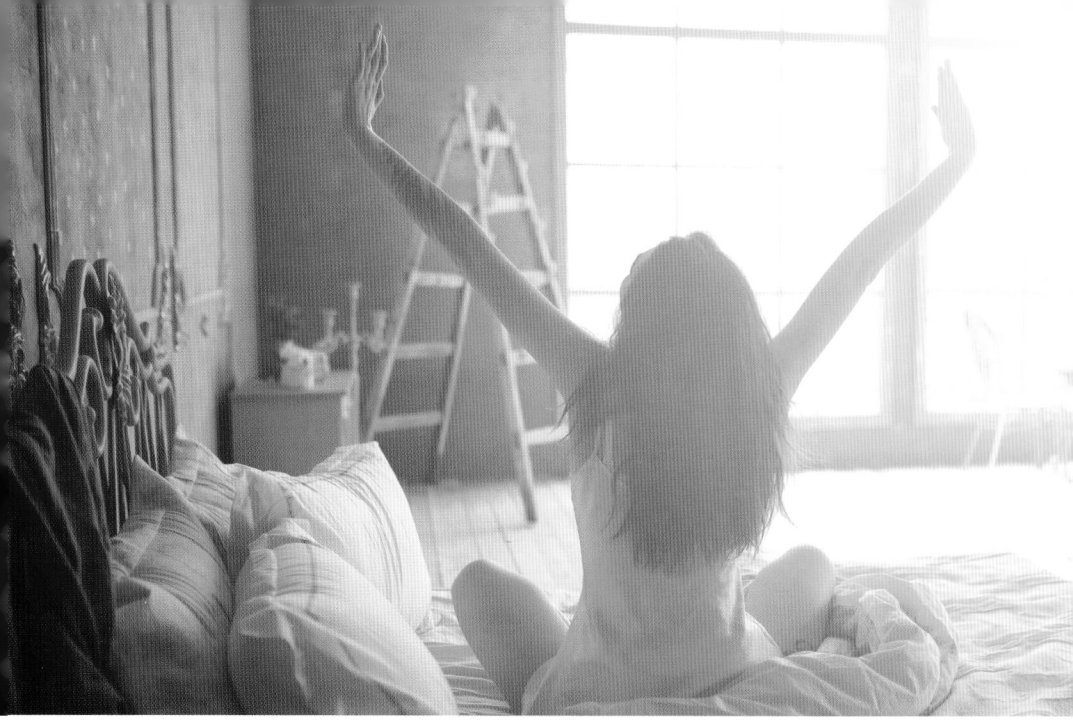

MR. WHARTON
...BRING ME A DREAM
How To Ensure A Great Night's Sleep

This is so obvious, but we all neglect it. By fitting in more and more into our lives, we neglect the most basic and useful of all things—sleep. If you need convincing that a good night of sleep is important, just google the science—the top sports trainers and coaches all insist that eight hours of sleep can help your body to heal and recover, and mentally you will have more energy and focus. I could tell you to try and get more sleep, but that's not helpful; you would just say to me, "Paul, honey, I know you mean well but you don't know how much I have going on."

I understand, so instead I am going to show you what I do every night to help myself go to sleep as quickly and smoothly as possible. Because the worst thing of all is when you lie there tossing and turning with your head full of stress (and then getting more stressed because you can't go to sleep).

Just like my advice for waking up each day, this only takes two minutes and I find it really helps to calm my mind after a challenging day.

Firstly, try to switch off as many devices as you can. If you have a phone, switch it off or put on airplane mode if you can. If you can't do that because you need to be able to answer a call if there's an emergency, then turn the volume down so that beeping messages won't wake you up but you can still be woken by a call. Secondly, try not to watch TV or read on the Internet just before you go to sleep. It takes your mind a little time to unwind and bright screens don't let you shut down properly.

Once you are in bed, lie flat on your back, again with your arms at the side or on your stomach. Close your eyes and take a couple of those deep breaths, in through the nose and out through the mouth. Just enjoy how it feels to be in bed. We spend our days rushing around, and you earned this rest, you earned this time to yourself. No one can bother you, this is your space now.

After those deep breaths, breathe normally and think back through the day, just like we did in the morning. Put it on fast forward and start with waking up, moving through the day, stopping at a few activities for just a few seconds. Keep breathing and just go through it all, without any judgment or feeling, until you reach the night and getting into bed.

Then take another deep breath and turn over or get comfortable for sleep, and just take a moment to remember that you deserve this rest and you earned the joy of being able to relax.

I do this every night and the goal is just to let go of the fears and worries of the day. Everything will be fine and nothing is going to change overnight. Any problems, any issues, can be dealt with tomorrow.

Nighty night . . .

IN THE ZONE

How To Improve Your Focus And Manage Nerves

Everyone has those incredible days when they're in the zone. We wake up with our brains firing, focusing in on each task and completing it in record time, managing to get through all those jobs we've been putting off. Nothing can stop us, even important meetings or dates feel effortless.

Sadly for most of us, those days are the minority. Mostly we lose minutes or hours by staring at a screen or reading the same words over and over, putting off important but annoying tasks. In short, we waste time because we can't get into a groove or zoom into whatever we need to be doing.

I hope one thing you've understood from this book is that I am trying to help you become more efficient and free up some of that precious time in your day. That's why the ability to focus is so important; if you can get your things done faster and be more efficient, you get more time in your day. So how do we do this?

Although everyone is different (you could be at school studying, taking care of a family, in an office typing memos, cooking, cleaning, or doing something totally different with your day), there is one universal thing that works for everybody— cut out distractions. Whatever you are trying to get done will go much faster and be better if you put away your phone, move to a quiet area away from people you know, and make sure you have set aside time where no one will bother you. Our brains can only handle a certain amount of stimulus, and if we have too much going on, it can't focus on the key thing at hand. So a very simple step is to . reduce the number of things that could distract you.

Now that you've got yourself some space and quiet, I want you to try something for me—sit up straight, close your eyes, roll back your shoulders, and take a couple of deep breaths in and out. As you do this, try to visualize what you are about to do, and see it being completed. Open your eyes and take another deep breath.

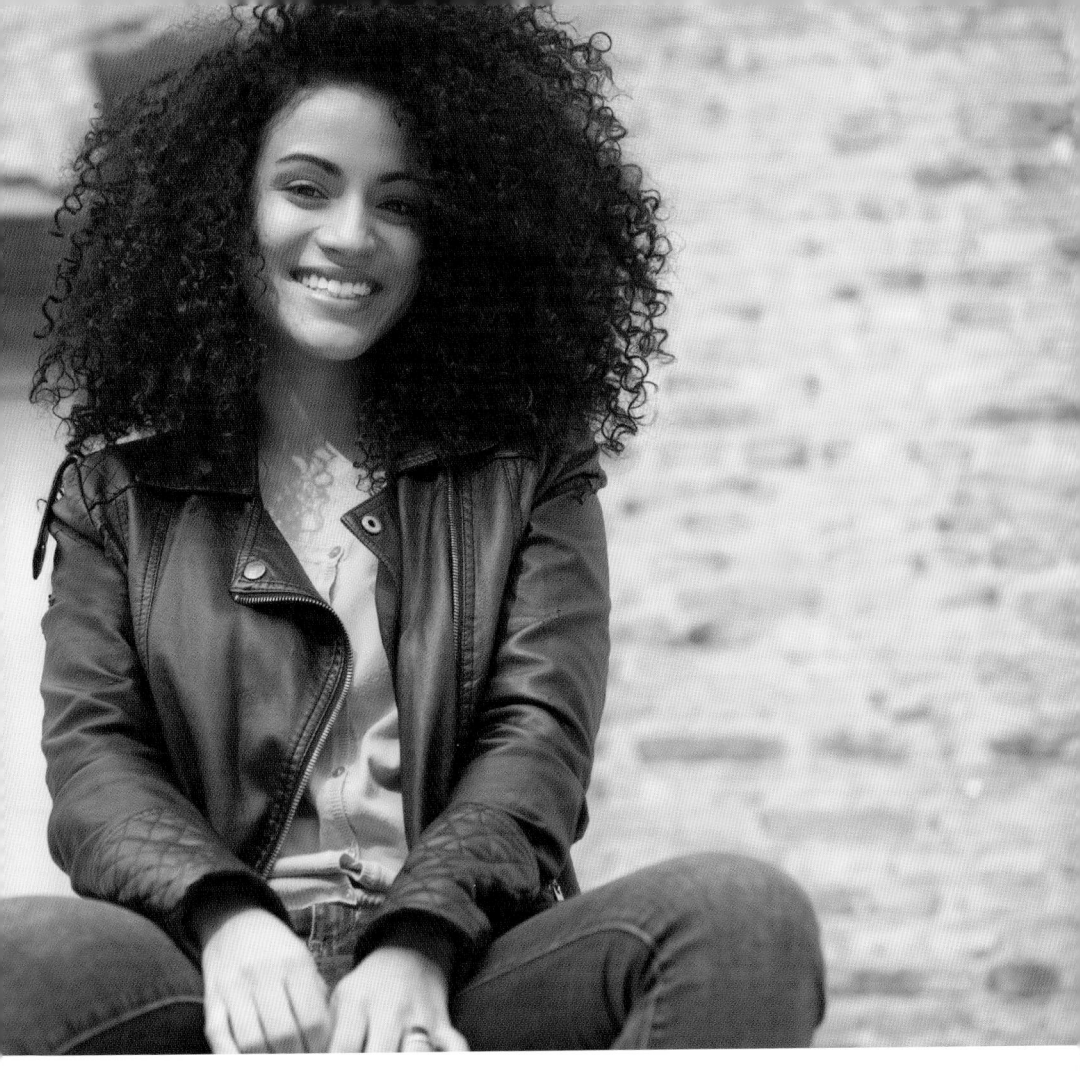

This is something I do when I need to focus; I find it helps me because I'm always carrying a million different ideas and conversations in my head. I need to bring myself into the moment, to put all that background noise out of my head and just focus on what I need to achieve. It's easy to forget just how much we carry around with us, so let it go. Stop thinking about the next job or the task after that—you'll get to all of them. But start with the issue at hand.

Now what if you have a big event, a job interview, important meeting, or an exam? The same rule applies: You need to bring yourself into the moment, but you also need to manage those nerves. Being nervous is not fun, and we've all made mistakes or performed worse than we should have just because we got tense. I know a lot of people who really struggle with this and it holds them back in life.

There is no one-size-fits-all option here because we all handle things differently, but I'd like to share a practice that I actually do, even if it sounds pretty strange—the "power pose." Remember how I told you earlier that when you feel yourself spiraling, you should sit up straight and smile? The power pose is a bigger version of that (in case you think this sounds dumb, you should look up a TED talk by Professor Amy Cuddy and see the science behind it).

A good friend of mine recently took a big exam and she was more nervous than I had ever seen her before. I passed on the same advice—before the exam, go to the bathroom and get into a cubicle so no one can see you, stand up tall and proud, and put your hands on your hips with your chest out and hold that for two minutes. I'm not going to tell you that this guarantees success—but it will probably make you feel better right before you go into that meeting or exam hall. It may give you that extra boost you need to put your nerves to the side and perform at your best. It certainly works for me.

I've been telling you about how to dress and take care of your skin and hair, but I'm not telling you to do those things for the benefit of other people. The way you perceive yourself affects how you perform and how others perceive you. If you believe that you are a strong, smart person, when you go to take on that task (whatever it may be), you will look like it and you will perform better.

So find yourself some space, put away the distractions, stay in the moment, take deep breaths, and fix that posture—now you can zone in and focus.

PAUL'S FINAL WORD

The #1 Rule (again)—Confidence

So, we have come full circle and I am so excited and happy that you have made this journey with me. I want to come back to the first and most important rule–be confident. This applies to every single chapter–in fact it applies to every single thing you do in your life.

Sometimes it feels like the whole world is trying to beat us down, telling us we're not good enough, showing us other people's successes and diminishing our own. Making us feel weak and worthless.

LET ME BE CLEAR— YOU ARE AMAZING.

Trust me on this one. I have met thousands of women through my work, my family, and my friends, and they are all remarkable, beautiful, and wonderful in their own unique ways. You are too. Sure, we can work on how to dress or improve our skin, but I don't want you to think that you are fixing flaws and weaknesses, you are just trying to improve a few things in your life (which is what we all should do every day). There is nothing wrong with you just as you are.

It is the most important lesson, and also the hardest . . .

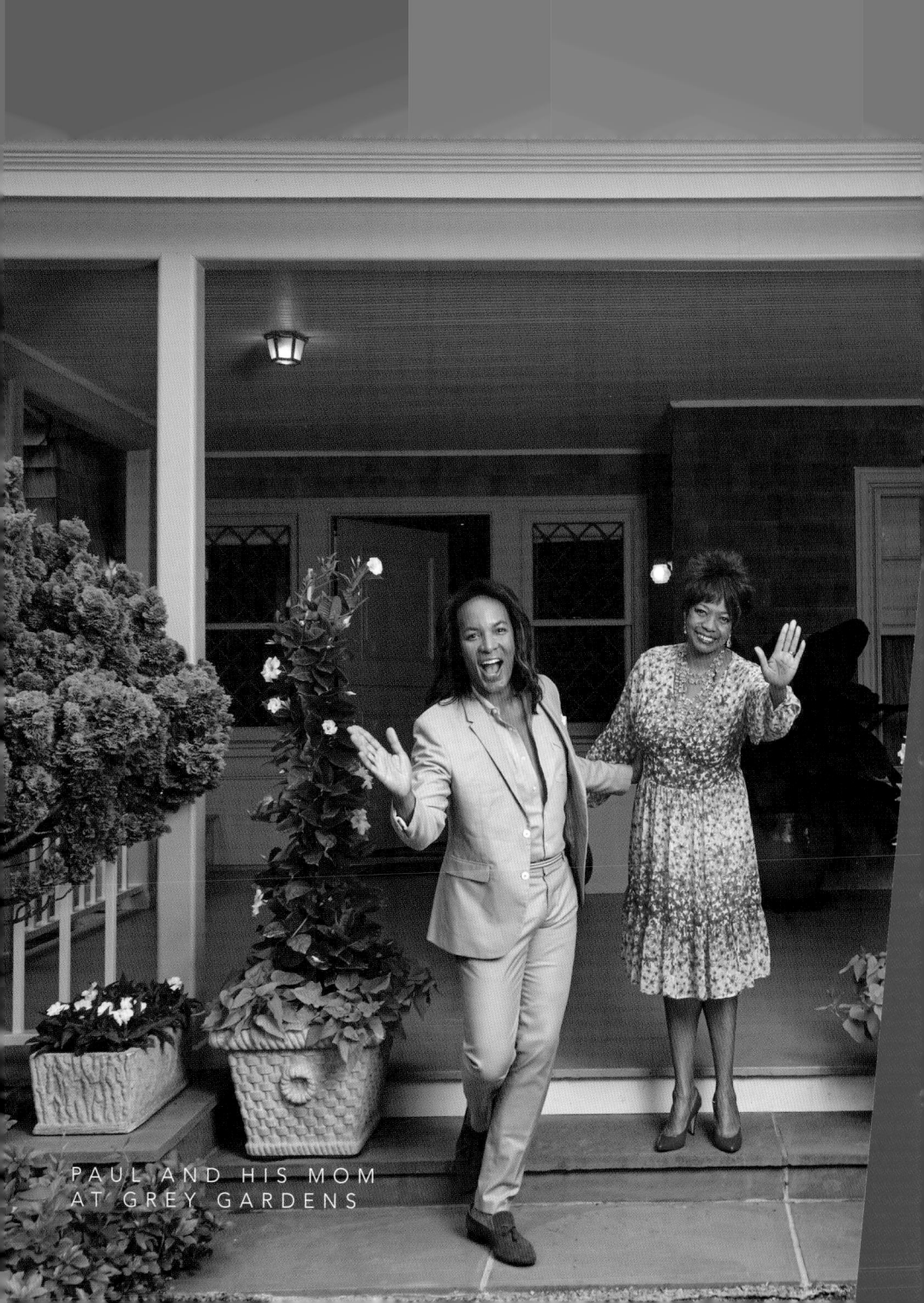

PAUL AND HIS MOM
AT GREY GARDENS

BE PROUD,
BE CONFIDENT
& BE HAPPY
IN YOURSELF.

YOU ARE
AMAZING

I hope you enjoyed this book and
I wish you all the very best of love, joy, and happiness as you

PULL IT ALL TOGETHER.

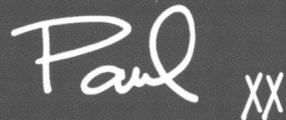

Pulling it all Together

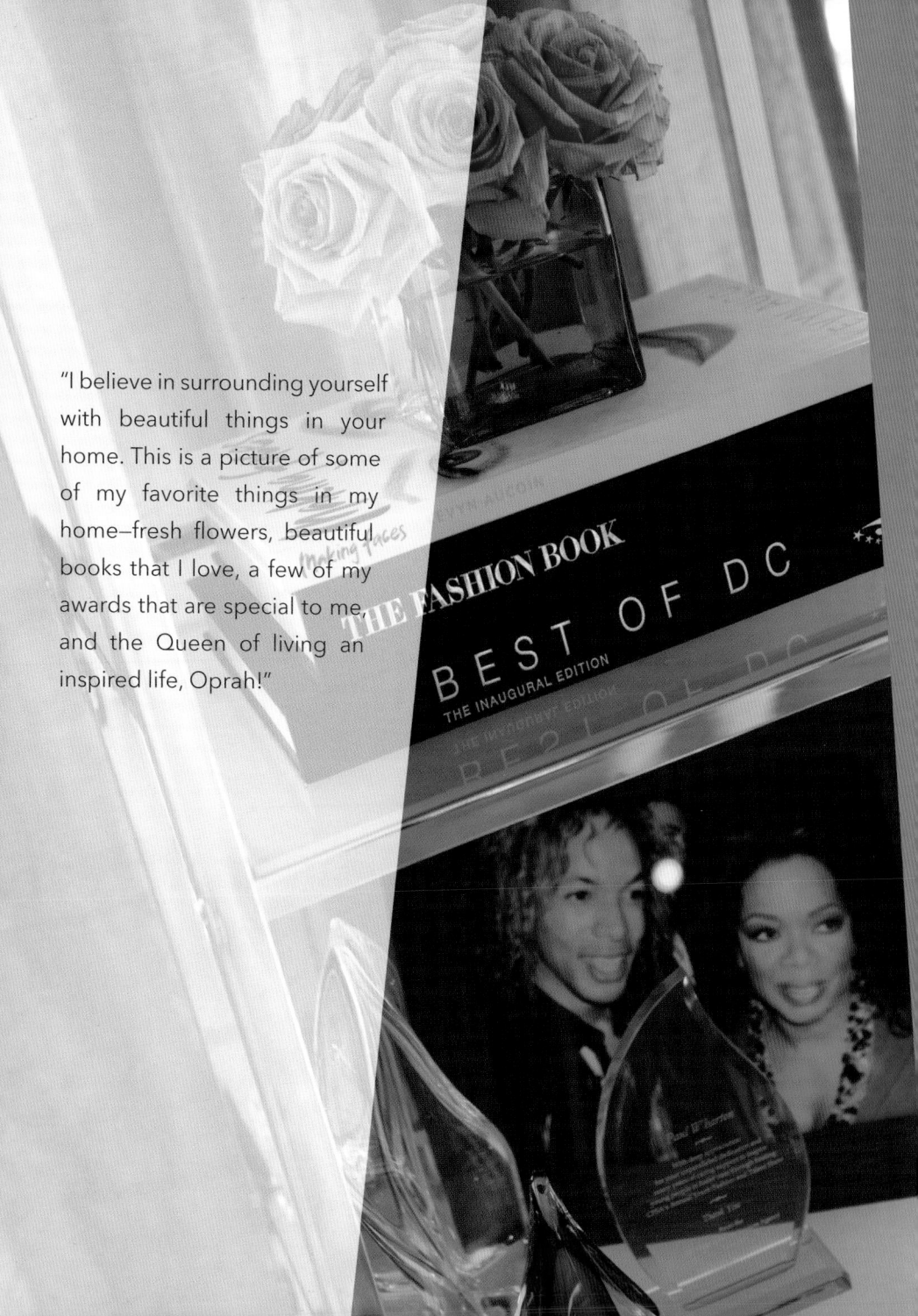

"I believe in surrounding yourself with beautiful things in your home. This is a picture of some of my favorite things in my home—fresh flowers, beautiful books that I love, a few of my awards that are special to me, and the Queen of living an inspired life, Oprah!"

INSPIRATION SCRAPBOOK

You might have heard of a technique called keeping a "Happiness Journal" or a "Gratitude Journal"—some people write down things that make them happy each day and this helps them to focus on the positives rather than the bad and gives them something to read through when they need to put a little pep in their step! I started doing something slightly different, I have an Inspiration Scrapbook where I put notes, pictures, mementos, and anything that has made me feel inspired or motivated. This helps me remember how lucky I am in life but also gives me a boost when I am working on a big project or taking on a new challenge. I can look and see the people and events that I've experienced along my journey and let the positive memories, and what that made me feel, propel me forward.

I would recommend you try something similar. It only takes a little time each week and you can do it in a physical scrapbook or use apps like Instagram to keep your journal.

FASHION
INSPIRATION

Betsey Johnson is just about the most unique individual I have ever known. Along with my mother, Betsey told me back in 2009 to write a book! Her honesty, compassion, loving spirit, raunchy talk, and ability to really zone in to whomever she is interacting with at the moment and listen with her ears, eyes, and heart, left an indelible mark on me. She's a fashion icon and an inspiration in my life. Hey Betsey, I wrote the book! I think that's cause for a cartwheel!

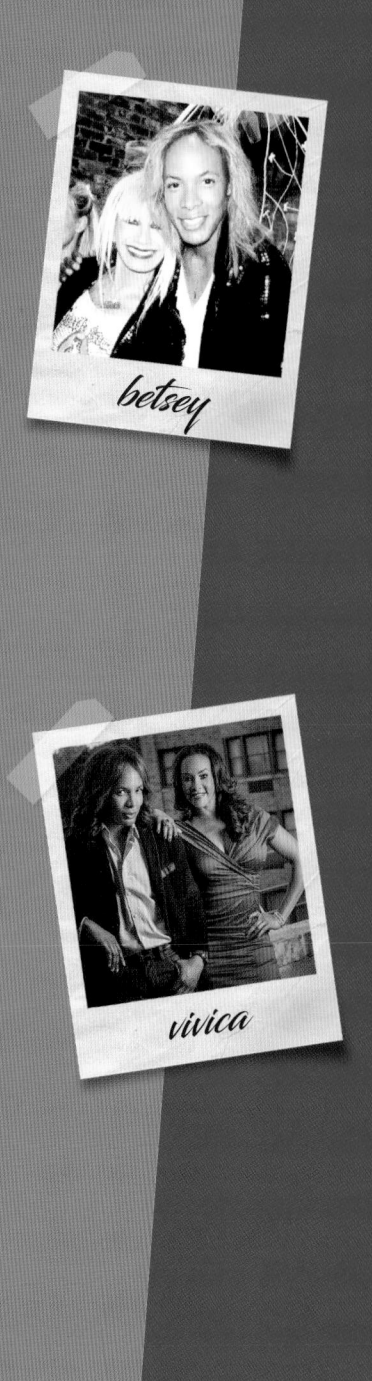

betsey

STAR
INSPIRATION

Before "Fashion Police" was on E!, BET launched a red carpet fashion commentary show called "Who Wore What." The show covered the hottest fashion on the red carpet and was hosted by Fonzworth Bentley, Vanessa Simmons, Vivica A. Fox and me! I knew Vivica casually for years but shooting "Who Wore What" and subsequently hanging out with Viv gave me a birdseye view into her genuine nature and kind heart. Vivica is not your everyday movie star! I respect her for her humility and intellect. Her quick wit and thoughtful advice. Let me sum it up by saying this: she's all heart, a woman that is full of love and light, but she will also "Set It Off" and that's why I love me some Vivica A. Fox!

vivica

MEDIA
INSPIRATION

Back in 2012, I set out to launch a new weekly talk show. I pulled the crew together but needed a popular television celebrity as my first guest to kick the show off and get sponsors interested. I barely knew Sherri Shepherd at the time but that didn't stop her from saying YES! Sherri gave me the best interview of my career and instantly became a good friend that I stay in touch with to this day. From her work as a co-host on "The View" to her thriving stand-up career and acting on network sitcoms, she remains humble, kind, and a woman that I respect and admire!

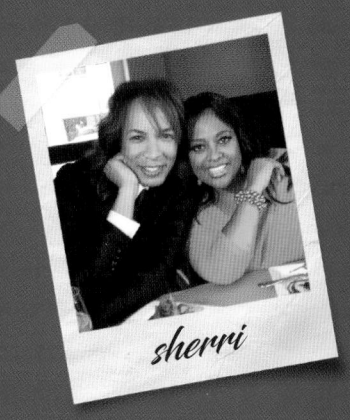

sherri

I was a part of the cast of "The Real Housewives of DC" on Bravo and boy, was that an experience I will never forget (did you see my birthday party?!). One of the best things to come from that reality roller coaster was getting to meet Andy Cohen and get a personal perspective on his work as a producer and television host. I certainly have my own style of interviewing, but I was able to grow my confidence in that area at least in part due to Andy's example. And, I love doing tequila shots with Andy Cohen! There, I said it! Mazel Andy!

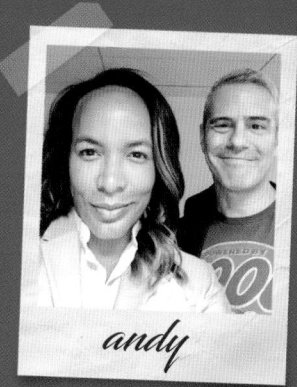

andy

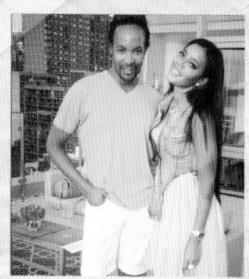

Angela #Calm

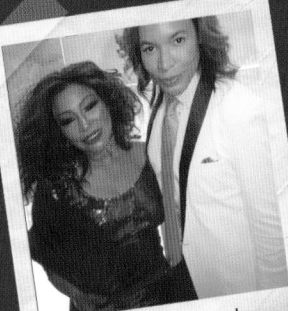

Chaka #Blessed

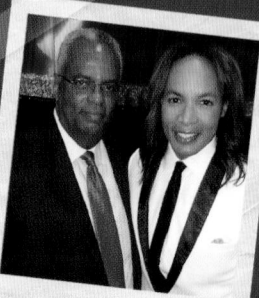

Dad #Love

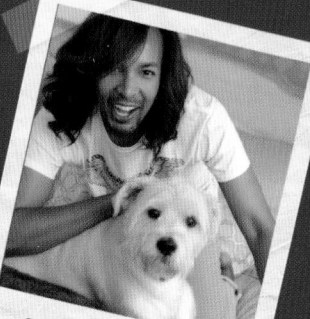

Oscar #Dedication

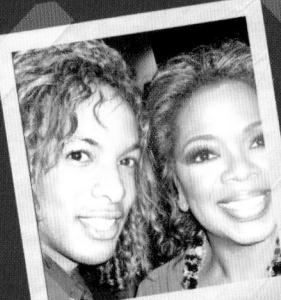

Oprah #Hope

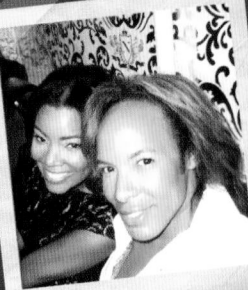

Gab #Spunk

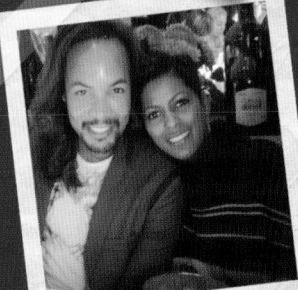

Tamron #Focus

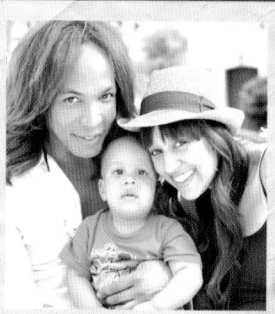

Tia #Serene

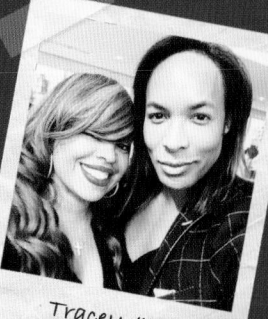

Tracey #Joy

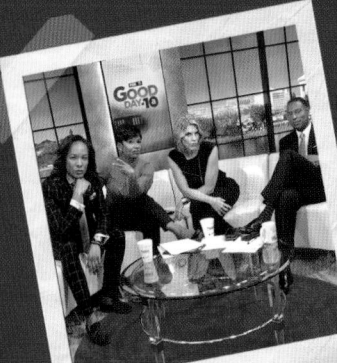

GoodDayDC
#Gratitude

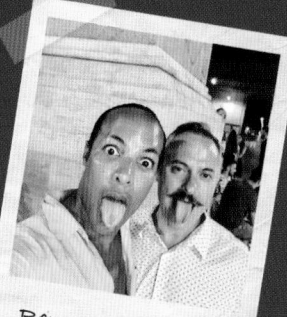

Renzo #Strength

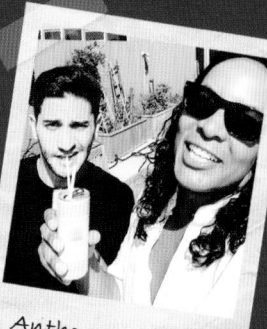

Anthony #Creative

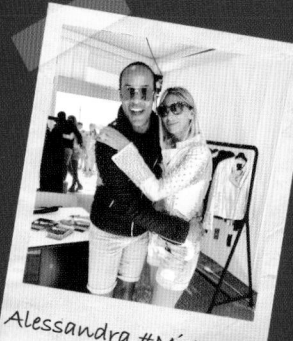

Alessandra #MiAmore

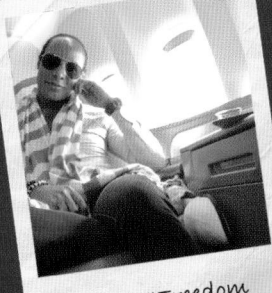

Travel #Freedom

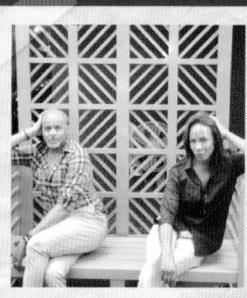

Timothais #Adventure

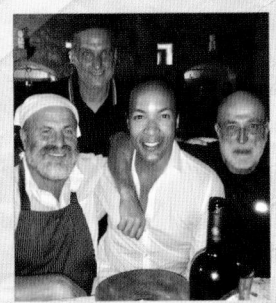

Fernando #Miraculous

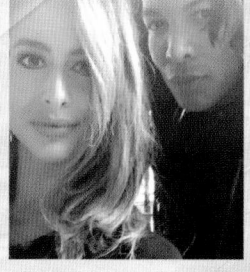

Erika #Loyal

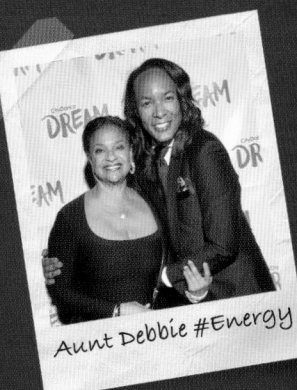

Aunt Debbie #Energy

@paulwhartonstyle

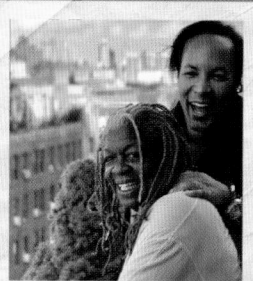

Jemaja #Integrity

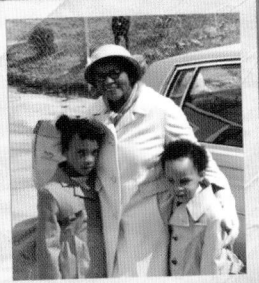

Grandmother Dorothy
#FirstLove

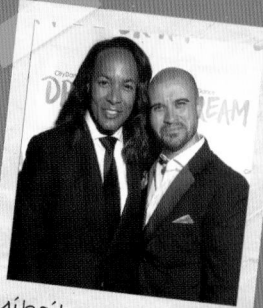

Mikail #Determination

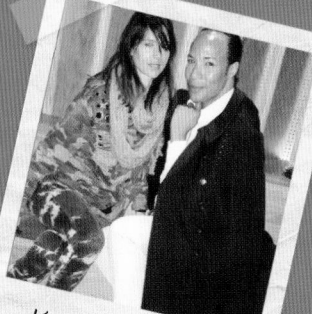

Karliin #Healthy

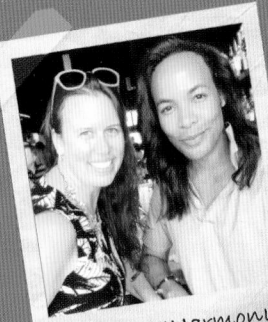

Mandy #Harmony

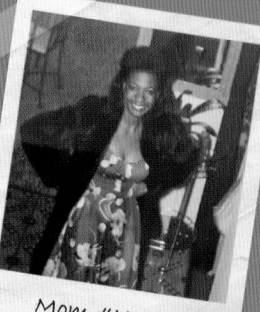

Mom #Happy

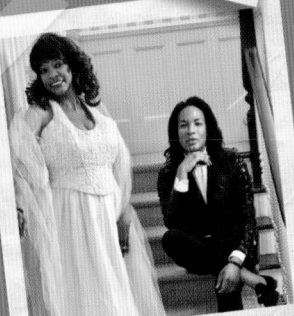

Grey Gardens #Believe

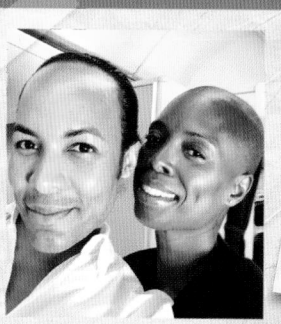

Sidra #Trust

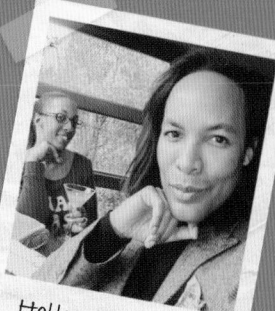

Holly #SisterLove

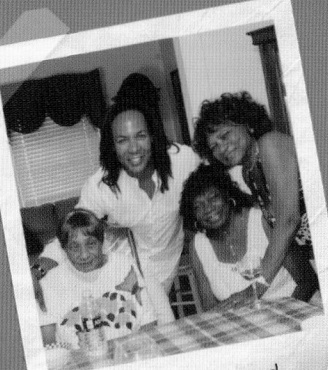

Roots #Cleveland

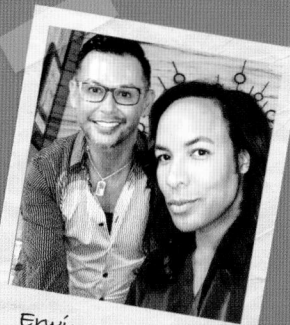

Erwin #Conquer

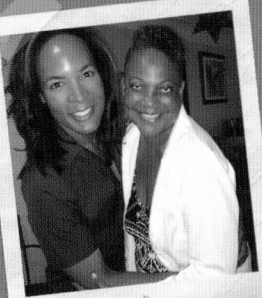

Karen #Humor

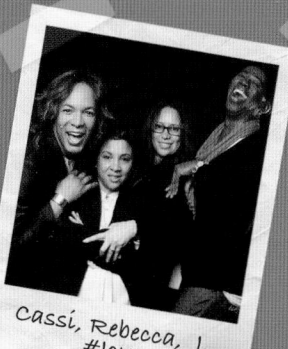

Cassi, Rebecca, J.
#Joy

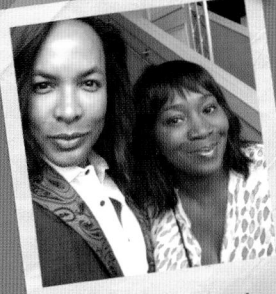

Bevy #Courage

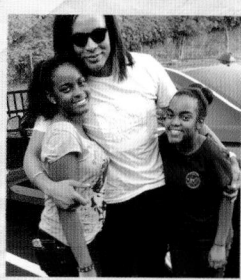

Nadia & Seana
#NieceLove

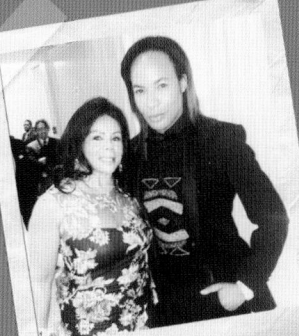

Marcia #Resilient

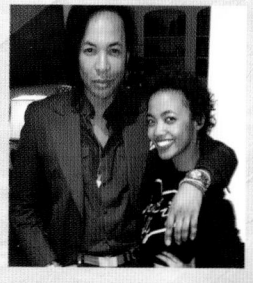

Anasia #Overcome

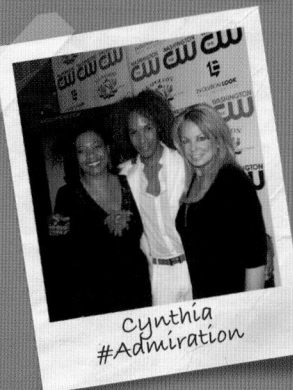

Cynthia
#Admiration

@paulwhartonstyle

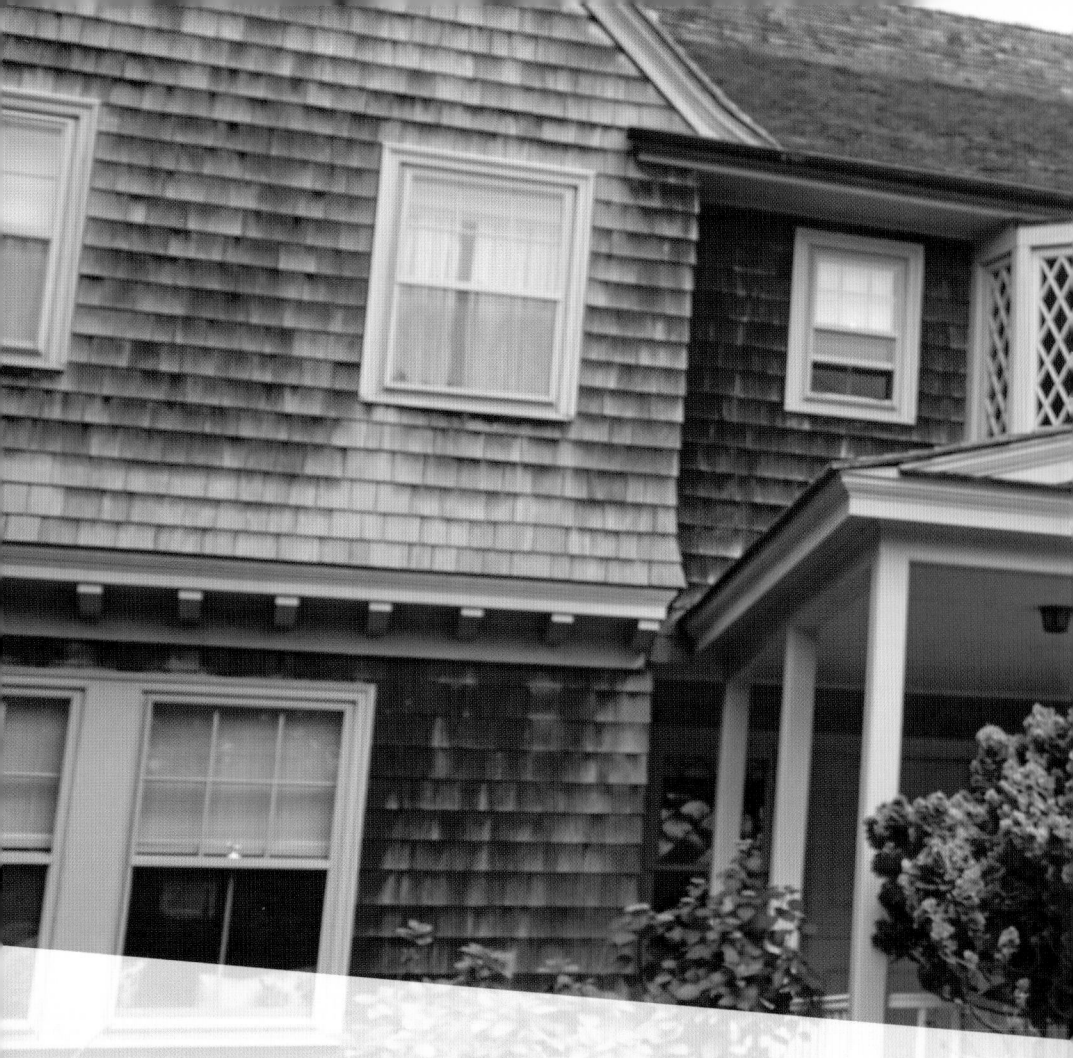

"This is the best thing to wear for today, you understand. Because I don't like women in skirts and the best thing is to wear pantyhose or some pants under a short skirt, I think. Then you have the pants under the skirt and then you can pull the stockings over the pants underneath the skirt. And you can always take off the skirt and use it as a cape. So I think this is the best costume for today."

—Edith (Little Edie) Bouvier Beale

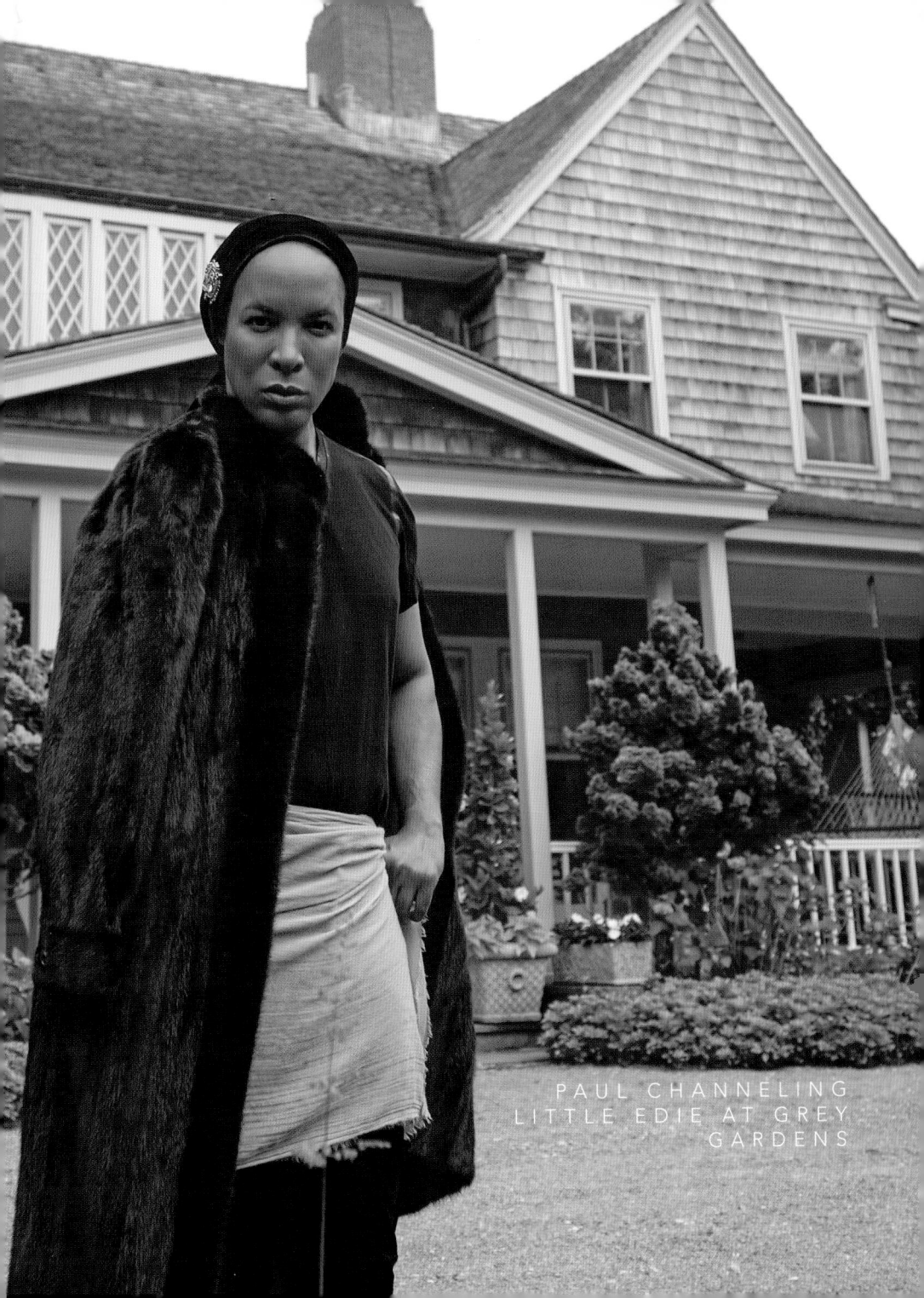

PAUL CHANNELING
LITTLE EDIE AT GREY
GARDENS

ACKNOWLEDGMENTS

This book would not have been possible without the following people helping me every step of the way. From the bottom of my heart, thank you:

To my publisher Tony Lyons and the entire team at Skyhorse Publishing for taking me on as a first time author. The "advance" truly did help to "advance" my confidence as an author. I appreciate your professionalism, flexibility, and patience.

To my editor Mikail Chowdhury. Mikail—who would've known that a chance meeting at a boozy bar in DC would bring together a bloke from London and a TV host from DC and make them into best mates? Working with you on this book has been one of the greatest joys of my life.

To my team at Paul Wharton Style—Creative Director/Designer Aidah Fontenot, we've been together for over ten years, and I think this is our best project to date. Thank you for your creativity, focus, and effort. I'm looking forward to the next ten years! To Traci Baker Jackson, my right hand woman—thank you. My glam squad Janelle Gladden, Kelly Simmons, Bouvier Davis, Lynne Wooden, LaNita LaDais, and Charlene Brown, thank you for keeping my look together. And thank you Taiana Hale, Diane Crawford, Paul Wharton Sr., and all of the other team members at PWS for your hard work and support.

To my family for your love and support—Mom, Dad, Holly, Chip, Renee, Anasia, Nadia, Seana, Grandmother Louise, Grandmother Dorothy, Aunt Flora, Aunt Barbara, Aunt Mary, Aunt Sharon, Aunt Vera, Uncle Tony, Uncle David, my stepbrothers Chris and Marty, all of my cousins and extended family in Cleveland. Wherever you are is home to me.

To my colleagues at Fox 5 DC—Jeff, Paul, Patrick, Maureen, Allison, Wisdom, Holly, and the rest of the team, thank you for greeting me with positive energy each morning we shoot Good Day DC, you're a phenomenal group of people.

And to my dearest friends—for a kid who started off a loner, you certainly have made coming into my own sweet. To the fabulous Rebecca James, Karen Williams, Gloria Harris, Dr. Charlotte Manning, Jemaja Selas, Tamron Hall, Sherri Shepherd, Timothais Thompson, Sidra Smith, Erika Gutierrez, Anthony Ferrara, Dr. Paul Ruff, Vivica Fox, Holly Wharton, Pari Bradlee, Pam Simpson, Bevy Smith, Miss Lawrence, Rob James, Marcia Dyson, Jocelyn Allen, Darnell Perkins, Sarah Fraser, Delband Vazir, Ginger Plummer Mair, Cynthia Wilson, Tracey Kearney, Lisa Bolden, Renzo Tomellini, Alessandra Grimoldi, Aja Shah, Maggie O'Neill, Wanda Durant, Erwin Gomez, Marko Thomas, Karliin Brooks, Charrisse Jordan, Tom Brown, Korie Mulkowski, Kathlene Buchanan, Jennifer Starling, Rey Gomez, Mary Barth, Cassi Caesar, Tomora Wright, Eric Eden, Scott Stewart, Brook Rose, Mandy Mills, David Getson, Donnell Kearney, Anthony Rodell, Charlotte Reid, and all of the other wonderful people that I call on and that call on me, day or night. We have each other's back and that means so much to me. Your support helped make this book possible. I love you all!

Cover: Photo by Chris Mills

p. iv: Photo by Barry Harley at Grey Gardens

p. viii: Photo by Barry Harley at Grey Gardens

p. ix: Photo by Jefry Andres Wright, Makeup LaNita LaDais | Hair Charlene Brown

p. 9: Photo by Fadil Berisha

p. 20: Photo of Wanda Durant by Barry Harley | Hair by Charlene Brown

p. 23: Photo by Chris Mills

p. 39: Photo of Tisha Hyter by Jefry Andres Wright

p. 46: Photo by Barry Harley

p. 54: Photo of Sidra Smith by Derek Blanks | Makeup by Saisha Beechem

p. 85: Photo by Jefry Andres Wright

p. 90: Photo by Chris Mills

p. 96: Photo by Chris Mills

p. 111: Photo of Tomora Wright by Jefry Andres Wright | Hair by Charlene Brown |
Makeup by LaNita LaDais

p. 114: Photo by Aidah Fontenot

p. 131: Photo by Tamu McPherson

p. 135: Photo by Aidah Fontenot

p. 140: Photo by Barry Harley

p. 145: Photo by Barry Harley

p. 158: Photo by Barry Harley